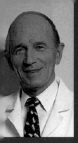

DR. KENNETH H. COOPER'S
ALL-NEW PLAN TO LOWER
CHOLESTEROL WITHOUT DRUGS

Controlling
Cholesterol
the
Natural Way

Eat Your ~~~~~~~~ th

New Breakt~~~~~~~~ eries

D0048177

KENNETH H. COOPER, M.D., M.P.H.

New York Times bestselling author of *Controlling Cholesterol*

Other books by
Dr. Kenneth H. Cooper

THE AEROBICS PROGRAM FOR TOTAL WELL-BEING

CONTROLLING CHOLESTEROL

OVERCOMING HYPERTENSION

Available wherever
Bantam Books are sold

BANTAM BOOKS

ISBN 0-553-58210-0

9 780553 582109

US $7.99 / $11.99 CAN

50799

S

Improve Your Cholesterol Profile the Natural Way

If you have a cholesterol problem, your primary objective should be to find a way to control your blood fats *without* drugs—as quickly as possible. Because functional foods are such great incentives for launching a successful, full-scale cholesterol-lowering program, I've included them in the first two steps of my all-new plan to lower your cholesterol.

Step 1: Reduce your total cholesterol by *10 percent* or more and your "bad" LDL cholesterol by *14 percent* or more by eating recommended daily servings of a designed functional food, such as Benecol or Take Control.

Step 2: Reduce your total cholesterol by *5 percent* with a traditional functional food, such as a cereal with high quantities of psyllium.

Step 3: Reduce your total cholesterol by *15 percent* or more with a low-fat, low-cholesterol diet.

Step 4: Raise your "good" HDL cholesterol by *10 percent* or more through regular endurance exercise.

Step 5: Lower your total cholesterol by *5 percent* for every 5 to 10 pounds you lose in excess body weight.

Step 6 (if necessary): Lower your total cholesterol by *25 percent* or more, and your "bad" LDL cholesterol by *30 percent* or more with statin drugs.

—Dr. Kenneth H. Cooper,
from *Controlling Cholesterol the Natural Way*

CONTROLLING CHOLESTEROL

THE NATURAL WAY

Eat Your Way to Better Health with New Breakthrough Food Discoveries

Kenneth H. Cooper, M.D., M.P.H.

Bantam Books

NEW YORK / TORONTO / LONDON / SYDNEY / AUCKLAND

Controlling Cholesterol the Natural Way
A Bantam Book / August 1999

All rights reserved.
Copyright (c) 1999 by Kenneth H. Cooper and William Proctor.

ISBN 0-553-58210-0

Published simultaneously in the United States and Canada

Bantam Books are published by Bantam Books, a division of Random House, Inc. Its trademark, consisting of the words "Bantam Books" and the portrayal of a rooster, is Registered in U.S. Patent and Trademark Office and in other countries. Marca Registrada. Bantam Books, 1540 Broadway, New York, New York 10036.

PRINTED IN THE UNITED STATES OF AMERICA

OPM   20   19   18   17   16   15

Contents

Acknowledgments

In addition to overseeing fundamental medical research at the Cooper Institute for Aerobics Research and pursuing an extensive medical practice as founder of the Cooper Clinic in Dallas, I also frequently find myself exploring new scientific and medical frontiers in my books. To communicate effectively and accurately with the general public, I often have to "get up to speed" in new areas of investigation—and this book is no exception.

As with my previous Bantam bestseller, *Controlling Cholesterol,* I have relied on the research and advice of a number of the world's leading blood lipid experts. These include two colleagues who are "close to home" in Dallas: Scott M. Grundy, M.D., Ph.D., director of the Center for Human Nutrition, University of Texas Southwestern Medical Center at Dallas; and Dr. Ishwarlal Jialal of the University of Texas Southwestern Medical Center at Dallas.

In addition, I am grateful for the contributions of scientists at other research facilities elsewhere in the United States and abroad—especially those who have done the recent groundbreaking research with "nutriceuticals," or "functional foods." As you'll see, these products are specially designed foods that have the power to prevent or heal cardiovascular diseases triggered by high or unbalanced cholesterol. Dr. Tu T. Nguyen, a leading endocrinologist and expert in blood lipids at the Division of

Endocrinology, Mayo Clinic in Rochester, Minnesota, has been quite helpful in explaining his research involving Benecol nutriceutical products, which are being marketed throughout the world by McNeil Consumer Healthcare, a unit of Johnson & Johnson. Dr. Ingmar Wester, vice president for research for the Raisio Group in Finland, has elucidated many of the scientific mysteries of the "plant stanol ester" process, which has made the production of Benecol possible.

The research staff at the Cooper Institute for Aerobics Research in Dallas, which has participated in the basic research involving the nutriceutical Benecol, has once again helped significantly in expanding our understanding of how this "functional food" works, especially in conjunction with medications.

Thanks are also due to the professionals at McNeil, as well as at the Kellogg Company, the Dutch-based Unilever's Lipton unit, Forbes Medi-Tech of Vancouver, and other organizations that are developing nutriceuticals that can be used to combat cholesterol problems.

In producing this manuscript, I am particularly grateful for the help of my longtime professional literary collaborator, William Proctor, who has worked with me on twelve other books since we met almost two decades ago. Bill and I have wended our way through a wide variety of fitness and preventive health issues—from the latest findings on aerobic fitness . . . to more traditional health concerns, such as hypertension and osteoporosis . . . to rather controversial topics, such as antioxidant supplements . . . and finally to our current topic, nutriceuticals. The proper role of nutriceuticals for the average patient will almost certainly dominate scientific discussions and research related to preventive medicine well into the next millennium.

Although our relationship has focused primarily on translating difficult scientific and medical concepts into understandable, readable language for the general reader, Bill and I have also become good friends—and have even found time in the midst of our labors to negotiate some rather difficult Colorado trails on mountain bikes.

The Book of Proverbs says, "Without consultation, plans are frustrated, but with many counselors they succeed" (Prov. 15:22). As much as any human being, I've been blessed with marvelous advisers, and the most important adviser in my publishing efforts over the past three decades has been my good friend and literary agent, Herbert M. Katz. Herb and his business partner and wife, Nancy B. Katz, have gone far beyond the role of traditional agents, as they have entered into the creative process, made helpful editing suggestions, and done a remarkable job in arranging for the sale of my books in more than forty languages.

My secretary and administrative assistant, Cynthia Grantham, has become increasingly important in serving as my "point person" in managing the ever-more-complex challenges posed by my international travel schedule and my burgeoning responsibilities at our home base in Dallas. Her understanding of the capacities of the computerized management of documents and e-mail transmissions has made my research and publishing efforts much easier and more efficient.

The support of the publishing and editorial staff at Bantam Books has been superb. Bantam president and publisher Irwyn Applebaum has inspired all of us with his confidence and commitment to this project. Without his vision this book would never have been possible.

Our editor, Robin Michaelson, has gone above and beyond the call of duty with her expert and insightful editing. Her enthusiasm and energy have been infectious—and have sustained us through multiple deadlines and the many demands of the editorial process.

Finally, my wife Millie has once again provided the

support and understanding at home that have enabled me to make it through another demanding literary endeavor, with all the attendant deadlines, late hours, and exhausting work.

My earnest hope—which I know is shared by all those who have supported me in this enterprise—is that as you read this book, you will find helpful guidance that will improve your health, and perhaps even save your life.

Kenneth H. Cooper, M.D., M.P.H.
Dallas, Texas

*To the research scientists and physicians
who are pushing back the frontiers of our
knowledge and increasing our understanding of
clinical application in the great war against
the cardiovascular killer cholesterol.*

Author's Note

In the scientific and popular literature, there is a variation in spelling of the operative word *nutriceutical*. Some scientists and writers use *nutriceutical,* as I do in this book. Others choose *nutraceutical.*

I prefer the *nutri-* version for several reasons. In the first place, these functional foods are without question a form of nutrition, and so it seems to me that a spelling that reflects this connection is appropriate.

Second, there is a strong linguistic argument for *nutriceutical.* The root for the English word *nutrition* is the Latin verb *nutrire,* which means "to nourish, suckle, or sustain." Related Latin words include *nutrimen* and *nutrimentum,* both of which are translated "nourishment."

Third, I can find no persuasive etymological precedents or arguments for the *nutra-* variation. As a result of these considerations—and despite the possibility that popular usage may eventually cause another spelling to prevail—I have chosen to use the *nutriceutical* spelling throughout this book.

Although I use real names whenever possible in my books, the demands of doctor-patient confidentiality and also privacy for those involved in research studies must often take precedence. Without this approach, I would be unable to present the full range of useful medical information that will help you achieve maximum lowering and balancing of your cholesterol. As a result, I have often changed the names or personal characteristics of patients and participants in research studies.

Note: Fitness, diet, and health are matters which necessarily vary from individual to individual. Readers should speak with their own doctor about their individual needs before starting any new diet or exercise program. Consulting one's physician is especially important if one is on any medication or already under medical care for any illness.

1

A Cholesterol Revolution?

More than ten years ago, I joined forces with other medical leaders in a revolution that has exploded into the consciousness of the general public—a revolution that has required us to confront head-on the lethal danger posed by cholesterol to the human heart and blood vessels. Through my bestseller *Controlling Cholesterol,* published in 1988, I was able to share insights from my own three decades of clinical work with cholesterol with millions of readers around the world.

Today, the revolution roars on. We now have learned that we can exert powerful control over cholesterol in natural ways that no one ever anticipated—through *functional foods,* or *nutriceuticals,* the terms now commonly used for table foods that have been specially designed to heal and prevent disease.

As chairman of the Cooper Institute for Aerobics Research, I elected to approve and supervise clinical trials on how certain functional foods behave in relation to harmful LDL cholesterol, beneficial HDL cholesterol, and other components of the blood lipid profile.

These and related research projects—at such far-flung

centers as the Mayo Clinic, the University of Helsinki, McGill University in Montreal, and the University of British Columbia—have broken much new ground. The startling findings have convinced those of us directly involved in the investigations that it is indeed possible to "eat your way to good health."

Yet what continues to amaze me is just how many of my conclusions in *Controlling Cholesterol* have *not* changed—even though much of our understanding about the operation and treatment of cholesterol *has* changed.

What Has Changed—and What Hasn't

What has changed on the cholesterol scene in the past ten years? A detailed answer will emerge in upcoming chapters, but here are some of the highlights:

- **Functional foods are revolutionizing our treatment strategies.** Now it's so much easier to control cholesterol naturally, without having to resort to medications.

- **Our understanding of "normal" total cholesterol has changed.** Ten years ago "normal" total cholesterol for an adult in the middle or older years would have been a reading below 235 to 240 mg/dl. Today acceptable total cholesterol is a measurement below 200.

- **Total cholesterol has taken a backseat to various cholesterol subcomponents.** I can still remember when many labs provided only one cholesterol number for a blood test—total cholesterol. Patients and physicians had to request specifically a reading on the important subcomponents—such as the "bad" LDL (low-density lipoprotein), the "good" HDL (high-density lipoprotein), and the ratio of total to HDL cholesterol.

Today every competent lab automatically reports these subcomponents because now we finally understand the serious danger posed both by low HDL cholesterol and by high LDL cholesterol.

● **Triglycerides—blood fats related to cholesterol—have assumed increasing importance as a cardiovascular risk factor.** Among other things, high levels of triglycerides are now regarded as a strong and independent predictor of the future risk of a heart attack—especially when total cholesterol levels are also high.

● **More attention is being paid to treating the cardiovascular concerns of women—especially those who have moved past menopause.** Although I warned in *Controlling Cholesterol* that postmenopausal women would lose the protection of estrogen and would become more vulnerable to heart disease, research into this subject was sparse ten years ago. Now we know that it's as essential to evaluate and treat women as it is to treat men.

● **Antioxidants—especially vitamins E and C—are assuming increasing importance in cholesterol-control programs.** Ten years ago the terms *antioxidant* and *free radical* were largely unknown to the general public or to practicing physicians. Today antioxidant vitamins have become an integral part of preventive medicine— and a powerful tool in controlling cholesterol the natural way.

- **More than ever, we are making use of what I call the Compound Effect in treating cholesterol.** This technique can reduce drug doses or even eliminate the need for them altogether. With this strategy (which I describe in detail in chapter 5) you begin with one approach to lowering cholesterol, such as functional foods, and then add a second approach, such as a low-fat diet. If necessary, you can add still another treatment, such as one of the new "statin" drugs.

    The combination of two or more of these treatments produces an exponential effect in controlling cholesterol, above and beyond what we've witnessed in the past—and typically limits the need for medications.

- **Noninvasive computer-imaging devices have taken much of the guesswork out of diagnosing clogged arteries—and are dramatically changing treatment strategies.** These new diagnostic techniques—which have been validated by several important studies published in major medical journals—are just emerging as a tool for practicing physicians in the United States and abroad. But the new technology, which is now available at the Cooper Clinic, has taught us that it's often not necessary to treat high total cholesterol with drugs—*if* a computer-imaging diagnosis plus a stress test indicate no coronary artery blockage.

    For example, ten years ago I would have prescribed medications for anyone with total cholesterol of 300 mg/dl (milligrams per deciliter). Today if a very low *calcification score* on computer imaging indicates no buildup of plaque (fatty deposits on arteries) and the treadmill stress test is normal, I wouldn't recommend drugs. Instead I would put the person on a cholesterol-lowering functional food regimen.

Yet even though many things have changed, many have remained the same. In reevaluating *Controlling Cholesterol*, I found that:

- A *low-fat, low-cholesterol diet,* accompanied by endurance exercise, is still the best starting point for a program to control cholesterol successfully.

- *Saturated fats,* such as those contained in butter and whole-milk products, continue to be a major dietary villain—and have been joined by *trans fats,* or those produced in the hydrogenation process during commercial manufacture of many foods.

- *Monounsaturated fats*—such as those found in olive and canola oil—continue to be the dietary fats of choice because, as Dr. Scott Grundy's research has demonstrated, they are associated with lower cardiovascular risk.

- *Obesity* is still as dangerous to your cardiovascular health and cholesterol levels as we believed ten years ago.

- *Stress* can upset a healthy blood cholesterol balance as much today as in the past.

- There is still a clear *correlation between aerobic exercise and higher levels of "good" HDL cholesterol*—for both men and women.

- The *statin drugs* were just coming into their own when I had the opportunity, in *Controlling*

Cholesterol, to introduce them to a much broader segment of the general public. Now, when medications are required, statins are the treatment of choice—and many more of them are available.

So we made a good start in dealing with the dangers of blood fats back in 1988, and considerable progress has been made since then. But most important, the message is getting across both to the medical community and to the general public—even though public awareness has sometimes been slow in coming.

We Finally Get It: Cholesterol Is Dangerous!

Research is one thing, but public awareness is another. During the 1970s even practicing physicians were slow to grasp just how dangerous cholesterol could be. At the Cooper Clinic, we certainly tested for cholesterol levels in those early days. But the meaning of the blood test results was still unclear because we couldn't attach a particular cholesterol measurement to a definite level of risk.

But gradually, as more research came in, we caught on. Other scientists pinpointed problems with certain subcomponents of cholesterol—such as too much "bad" LDL (low-density lipoprotein) or too little "good" HDL (high-density lipoprotein).

Much of the important basic research about the dangers of cholesterol was finally in place in the 1980s, but public and even physician awareness was slow in crystallizing. Even as *Controlling Cholesterol* was hitting the bookstores in 1988, many practicing doctors didn't put much stock in the warnings about the dangers of cholesterol.

I still recall with some sadness a discussion that occurred at a party organized in 1988 by a man suffering from heart disease. His physician, an invited guest, argued strenuously and mockingly with one of my colleagues against the "fashionable but misguided" idea that elevated cholesterol could be linked to heart attacks and a shorter life.

The doctor had studied the professional literature to some extent and could handle the then-strange terminology, such as *lipoprotein* and *total-to-HDL-cholesterol ratio* with a degree of facility. At the end of the debate, he was holding his own, and I'm sure he left with a sense of satisfaction that he had corrected some of the "bad information" that was floating about.

Unfortunately, about a year later, his patient, who had organized the party, suffered a massive heart attack. Shortly afterward the man died, the victim of atherosclerosis—the clogging or "hardening" of the arteries that results from the buildup of plaque, which is caused by the oxidation of "bad" LDL cholesterol.

Despite such resistance by some members of the medical community, the true danger of high cholesterol has gradually registered—in part as a result of pressure from savvy patients, and in part because of increasing knowledge among physicians. In fact, the scientific support for the cholesterol threat had become quite clear to most physicians by the beginning of the 1990s.

Among other things, as I've already suggested, investigators had accumulated overwhelming evidence that the higher your total cholesterol—especially at levels above 200 mg/dl—the higher your risk of heart disease. One widely accepted way of expressing this danger is that over a period of several decades, for every one percent rise of cholesterol above 200 (or just 2 mg/dl), the risk of coronary heart disease rises by 3 percent.

Also, it has become generally accepted among leading researchers that for patients *without* a history of cardiovascular disease, "bad" LDL cholesterol should be lower than 130. And we have learned that those *with* a history of heart or vessel disease should keep their LDL below 100. Also, the ratio of total to "good" HDL cholesterol should be 4.2 or lower for men and 3.0 or lower for women.

Unfortunately, many of these new findings are only now becoming known among many practicing physicians—in part because the flood of new research findings sometimes obscures the most important new treatment strategies that are now available.

A Snapshot of the Current Cholesterol Threat

Physicians "in the trenches"—including those treating people every day with out-of-control cholesterol—are eager, if not desperate, to find new ways to lower their patients' risk. They are open to improved treatment techniques, and they are also optimistic because of how much their patients have been helped by the new statin drugs and other recent breakthroughs.

Just consider the dramatic drop in cholesterol levels over the last three decades. The total cholesterol level for the average American adult declined from 220 mg/dl in 1960, to 213 in 1978, and to 205 in 1990, according to Dr. James Cleeman, coordinator of the National Cholesterol Education Program (NCEP). (See *Lipid Management,* vol. 1, no. 2, Fall 1996, pp. 1ff.)

Furthermore, only about 20 percent of Americans today have significantly high levels of cholesterol—or measurements of 240 or above. This compares with 26 percent in this "high risk" to "very high risk" category in 1978.

Even more reassuring, almost half of Americans—49 percent—now have what Dr. Cleeman calls "desirable" total cholesterol levels lower than 200 mg/dl. In contrast, 44 percent had readings this low in 1978.

One reason for the improvement is that public awareness of the cholesterol threat is up. Now three-quarters of Americans have had their total cholesterol level checked at least once—a great improvement over the 35 percent who had undergone a cholesterol test in 1983. Also, 49 percent of American adults—about 85 million people—now know their cholesterol levels, as compared with a mere 3 percent in 1983.

Obviously, we've made progress in broadening public awareness and treatment. But even with these encouraging findings, it's clear that we still have a long way to go—and good reason to beware of complacency.

The Dangers of Complacency

To begin with, more than half of all Americans—or 51 percent—still have cholesterol levels above 200 mg/dl. Or to put it another way, nearly 100 million adults in the United States alone, or about half the adult population, don't meet national standards for a safe lipid level.

With such a threat looming over us, it's imperative that physicians and patients alike get those elevated cholesterol readings down to normal levels.

However You Do It, Get That High Cholesterol Down!

Why is it so important to lower your cholesterol? The simple answer: a longer life.

A five-year study published on November 16, 1995, in the *New England Journal of Medicine* provided what many scientists regard as proof that you can live longer by controlling your cholesterol. The Scottish investigators found that otherwise healthy middle-aged men—who ranged in age from 45 to 64 and whose total cholesterol was 250 to 300—reduced their overall death rate by one-fifth by taking a statin drug, pravastatin (brand name: Pravachol).

Specifically, by the end of the five-year period, those on the drug suffered 31 percent fewer nonfatal heart attacks, were 32 percent less likely to die of cardiovascular disease, and experienced a 22 percent drop in death rate.

A 1998 study, also published in the *New England Journal of Medicine,* confirmed that lowering cholesterol will lengthen life—but this time the subjects were men with a history of heart attacks or unstable angina (chest pains from a lack of blood flow to the heart).

The more than 9,000 participants, who ranged in age from 31 to 75 and had total cholesterol levels from 155 to 272, were given pravastatin (Pravachol) and then monitored for more than 6 years. The researchers found that those undergoing this drug therapy—in contrast to a placebo group that received no drugs—suffered fewer deaths from coronary heart disease or from other causes. (See *New England Journal of Medicine,* vol. 339, Nov. 5, 1998, pp. 1349–57.)

Clearly, lowering elevated cholesterol will save lives, but it's even more desirable to achieve these results *without* drugs. And now we are in a position to take advantage of perhaps the most important nondrug treatment for cholesterol ever discovered. This new, natural strategy promises to improve the health of countless patients, including one I'll call Marie, who first came through the Cooper Clinic almost ten years ago.

A Woman Named Marie

Marie—a public relations executive who labored in the high-stress corporate environment of one of the world's largest cities—had taken time out from her busy schedule to travel thousands of miles to see us because she was deeply worried about her health—and especially about her out-of-control cholesterol.

Having studied my *Controlling Cholesterol*—which she bought after she noticed a risk chart from the book attached to a bulletin board in her own doctor's office—Marie decided that her best chance to get her blood lipids into shape would be to use the programs offered by the Cooper Clinic. In fact, she decided to spend her entire four-week annual vacation in the Dallas area in a concerted effort to improve her cardiovascular risk profile.

Then in her mid-fifties, Marie had been postmenopausal for a couple of years, and as a result she had lost the protection of estrogen against cardiovascular disease. According to her last blood test, her cholesterol levels were quite abnormal. (For a comparison, see the recommended levels in chart 1 on page 30.) Here's a summary of the results:

- Her total cholesterol was 320 mg/dl, or well into the very "high" range, far above the "acceptable" level of less than 200.

- Her "bad" LDL cholesterol was 252—again, in the extremely high-risk range and far above the "acceptable" LDL level of less than 130.

- Her "good" HDL cholesterol was reasonably normal at 56.

- Her ratio of total cholesterol to "good" HDL cholesterol—perhaps the best marker of cholesterol-related cardiovascular risk—was 5.7, or a very "high" risk reading and far above the "acceptable" level of 3.0 or below.

Marie was particularly worried because of her family history of cardiovascular disease—and with good reason. Her mother had died of a heart attack when she was about Marie's age. Her father had suffered his first *myocardial infarction,* or heart attack, when he was even younger, in his early fifties.

"I may be able to hold on a little longer because I've tried to watch my diet and weight more closely than my parents did," Marie observed. "But if genes and cholesterol mean anything, I could be in big trouble in the near future."

I could only agree with her assessment. But I did think she had a good chance to lower her risk to an acceptable level if she followed a wise treatment program.

Because I have always preferred prescribing drugs only as a last resort, our first line of attack on her cholesterol was to encourage her to make some cholesterol-lowering lifestyle adjustments—including changes in her dietary and exercise patterns. Fortunately, because she planned to be near our clinic for about a month and make regular visits to see our physicians and health care staff, we could monitor closely how she responded to these strategies.

Marie was close to her ideal weight—only about ten pounds over what I would have preferred. But because any extra body fat is often associated with elevated total and "bad" LDL cholesterol, I urged her to get rid of those extra pounds.

Fortunately, she had already been consuming a reasonably low-fat diet, so she was at least heading in the right direction in her food choices. According to a nutritional analysis of her meals, her total daily intake of fats represented 29 percent of her total calorie consumption.

But about 15 percent of those fat calories involved saturated fats—or the type that are most likely to promote high levels of blood cholesterol. So we recommended that she change her diet by taking in only about 20 to 25 percent of her daily calories in fat, with about 7 or 8 percent of her total calories coming from saturated fats.

Also, I asked her to focus more seriously on endurance exercise, which can be an important factor in raising levels of "good" HDL cholesterol. This is a particularly important consideration for several reasons.

For one thing, in a number of studies higher HDL levels have been associated with lower cardiovascular risk. Also, as the HDL rises, the ratio of total to HDL cholesterol drops—and that's another extremely important factor in lowering cardiovascular risk.

Marie had been walking at a moderate pace for 20-minute sessions about two days per week, and again, that was a good start. But I suggested that she increase her aerobic activity to four days per week, at 30 minutes per session.

She made some headway over the next three weeks. Her total cholesterol dropped to 285, her "bad" LDL cholesterol went down to 198, and her "good" HDL rose slightly to 57. These changes meant that her ratio of total to HDL cholesterol declined to 5.0.

These results still left her in the "high" risk ranges, but her blood-lipid profile was certainly better than when she had begun. Still, given her family history of heart problems, she needed to do more—and that meant I had to recommend cholesterol-lowering medications.

I prescribed one of the new lipid-lowering statin drugs, which usually lower both "bad" and total cholesterol without affecting the "good" cholesterol. Marie's blood cholesterol profile improved almost immediately: Her total cholesterol, "bad" LDL cholesterol, and ratio all dropped down to well within the normal ranges.

Unfortunately, Marie turned out to be one of those people who could not tolerate the statin drugs. Almost immediately she began to suffer from a form of myopathy, a degenerative muscle disease that causes weakness and fatigue. She could hardly get out of bed in the morning. Her energy levels fell to a point that was literally crippling.

Since her negative responses were so debilitating, we switched her to one of the bile acid sequestrants, which lower cholesterol using a different biological mechanism from that employed by the statins. But again, Marie experienced unacceptable side effects, including gastrointestinal upsets, nausea, and constipation.

When the time finally arrived for Marie to return home, we were *still* in a quandary about what long-term treatments to prescribe—an extremely frustrating state of affairs for me, since I'm accustomed to getting positive results with patients in her situation. Clearly, Marie needed to continue with the diet and exercise programs that she had started. But to get her lipids into an acceptable cholesterol range, she required medications. The question was *which* medications?

To see if the weakness and fatigue might abate somewhat over time as her body adjusted to the drugs, I recommended that Marie go back on the statin medication—at least for a few weeks. When she returned home, however, she reported that she simply couldn't function at work, and the rest of her life was on hold as well. I finally told her the only thing I could, which was that she should drop the statin and we would see what we could accomplish with other strategies.

We tried niacin. We increased her dietary restrictions and increased her exercise. These adjustments worked to some extent. But because of the side effects, she still couldn't tolerate large enough doses of any drug to be able to take her cholesterol into the range that I preferred.

Fortunately, Marie didn't give up—and her perseverance is about to pay off. With the advent of the new functional foods, her prospects for complete cholesterol control have improved significantly. Here is the way her program will now work *without any drugs at all,* as she begins to use cholesterol-lowering functional foods.

With the average results shown in various studies, she will be able to lower her total cholesterol from 285 to about 218. Her "bad" LDL cholesterol should drop from 198 to about 154, while her "good" HDL cholesterol will remain unaffected at 56. (There's even a possibility that a person's HDL cholesterol may increase with these nutriceuticals.)

With these changes Marie's measurements would fall well within the "borderline" category in chart 1 on page 30. Also, her all-important ratio of total to HDL cholesterol would go down to 3.89 (a figure calculated by dividing 218 by 56).

Remember, too, that we're talking about *averages* here. Some patients may enjoy lower decreases in cholesterol levels, but many others will benefit from reductions that are much greater than the average.

But even with just the average results, Marie will have a much healthier cholesterol risk profile, and a much better chance of avoiding cardiovascular problems such as heart attack or stroke. Furthermore, she will be in a position to take extremely small doses of one of the statin drugs—doses of 5 mg per day that will be unlikely to trigger the side effects she was experiencing before.

Marie, then, is a prime candidate to take full advantage of the new era of functional foods, which is about to change the lives of many patients with cholesterol concerns.

The New Era of Cholesterol-lowering Functional Foods

A decade ago functional foods that lower cholesterol didn't even exist—and most medical researchers had no idea that they were about to burst forth on the treatment horizon.

Yet now a spate of solid scientific studies—in such respected journals as the *New England Journal of Medicine, Circulation, Atherosclerosis,* and the *American Journal of Epidemiology*—have established that relatively small servings of these nutriceuticals can work wonders to lower cholesterol. Researchers have demonstrated conclusively that these nutriceuticals can reduce total cholesterol on average by 10 to 22 percent, and "bad" LDL cholesterol by 14 to 22 percent. Furthermore, a series of incontrovertible scientific investigations have shown that these significant reductions in cholesterol can occur in *only two to eight weeks, with no side effects!*

These results, which I have been observing personally as our clinical trials proceed at the Cooper Institute, have been evaluated and confirmed by such scientists as:

• Dr. Scott Grundy, director of the Center for Human Nutrition at the University of Texas Southwestern Medical Center, Dallas—widely regarded as the world's leading cholesterol researcher. (While he was director, his colleagues Dr. Michael S. Brown and Dr. Joseph L. Goldstein won the Nobel Prize for medicine for their work on "receptors," or protein strands in the liver and other tissues, which catch a deadly form of cholesterol that circulates in the bloodstream.)

• Dr. Tu T. Nguyen, a leading blood lipid expert at

the Division of Endocrinology, Mayo Clinic, Rochester, Minnesota; and

- Dr. Tatu A. Miettinen of the Department of Medicine, University of Helsinki.

Extensive and highly successful laboratory tests and clinical studies have encouraged several of the world's largest consumer goods companies to produce a variety of cholesterol-lowering functional foods for supermarket shelves—including spreads, salad dressings, and yogurts, sold under such brand names as Benecol and Take Control.

But as you'll see, this is just the beginning of the great story that is unfolding in the current revolution in cholesterol control.

Coming Attractions

In the following pages, we'll explore in great detail how the incredible new nutriceuticals can solve many different kinds of cholesterol problems—including, most likely, your own.

In chapter 2 you'll get a quick primer in cholesterol—how it works in your body and how to evaluate your own risk.

Chapter 3 will focus on the twin pillars of "lifestyle treatment"—diet and exercise. As in the past, these two mark the starting point for any successful strategy in cholesterol control.

Chapter 4 will provide you with important background information about how research into wood pulp, soybean extracts, and "ancient grains" has led to the cholesterol-lowering nutriceuticals now on your supermarket shelves.

In chapter 5, you'll get details about the all-important Compound Effect, one of most important innovations in cholesterol treatment in the last decade. Among other things, I'll introduce you to practical strategies for combining functional foods with diet, exercise, and when necessary, drugs.

The solid scientific support for the new "designed" functional foods, which contain special plant extracts, can be found in chapter 6. I highlight the landmark 1995 *New England Journal of Medicine* report by Finnish researchers on the power of functional foods with plant stanol esters.

In chapter 7, we'll turn to strategies for combining the functional foods with different drugs—and how doses can be reduced or even eliminated completely. One feature of this chapter, which many of my patients have found useful, is a detailed summary of the main drugs that are currently available—their operation in the body and their potential side effects.

In chapter 8, you'll find recipes and meal suggestions for the "best medicine you ever ate"—with some functional foods containing plant extracts and others offering soluble fiber.

The latest information available on the cholesterol-related cardiovascular problems of women will be reviewed in chapter 9. In particular we'll pay attention to the concerns of postmenopausal patients like Marie, who have lost the protection of estrogen.

In chapter 10, I've dared to take a look into the future and project what the "next step" may be in controlling cholesterol. There we'll explore not only the outlook for functional foods but also new treatment possibilities, diagnostic tools, and groundbreaking research on the chemistry of cholesterol.

You'll receive the latest "scoop" on vitamin and dietary supplements that relate to the control of cholesterol and the lowering of cardiovascular risk in chapter 11.

Finally, in chapter 12, I'll respond to questions that are commonly posed to me about cholesterol-related problems. Here are a few of the specific issues we'll explore:

- Can eating just one high-fat meal raise your risk of a heart attack?

- What other health benefits may lipid-lowering functional foods confer?

The cholesterol landscape is changing so quickly that you may feel it's nearly impossible to know exactly what strategies are best for treating your own blood lipids. In the following pages, I plan to unmask much of the mystery and confusion—and to use the nutriceutical revolution to get you well on your way to the completely natural control of your cholesterol.

2

Cholesterol 101

Cholesterol research involves some of the most complex molecular and biochemical issues in the history of modern medicine. But it's not necessary for you to become an amateur scientist to understand what you need to know to control your own cholesterol. All that's required is the simple "crash course" that I'm offering in this chapter. First you'll get a basic explanation of how cholesterol works in your body. Then I'll provide some guidelines for evaluating your own risk.

A Crash Course in How Cholesterol Works

Cholesterol may be the greatest enemy to the health of our heart and blood vessels—but it's also essential to life.

A whitish, waxy fat or *lipid,* cholesterol can be found throughout the body's blood and tissues. It plays a vital role in the formation of cell membranes and the production of certain hormones, such as steroid hormones in the adrenal glands and sex organs. Cholesterol also helps form bile acids in the liver, which aid in digestion in the small intestine.

So our objective in this book is *not* to wage an all-out war on cholesterol in an effort to eliminate it. Rather, we simply want to *control* this fat, in an effort to prevent high accumulations of cholesterol, or *hypercholesterolemia,* in the bloodstream.

Here's the problem: If too much cholesterol accumulates in the blood, the disease of *atherosclerosis* may occur—with a buildup of plaque on the artery walls and the eventual blockage of one or more vessels that transport blood to the heart. When the heart is deprived of blood and the oxygen that it carries, a heart attack results.

According to our best current scientific understanding, the cholesterol threat—which may be likened to a well-organized, rather sedate party gone haywire—arises this way:

The party begins in the liver, the large organ in the upper right part of the abdomen, which performs many essential functions, such as producing bile, metabolizing proteins, and purifying blood. The festivities then extend into your bloodstream and touch tissues and organs throughout your body.

The liver oversees the activities of several "party people," three of which are most important for our purposes:

Guest 1: Low-density lipoprotein (LDL) cholesterol

Guest 2: Triglycerides

Party Security Force: High-density lipoprotein (HDL) cholesterol

Each of these is a blood fat or lipid in molecular form, but they each have quite different personalities and characteristics. When they attend the party in your circulatory system in their proper numbers, as well-behaved, invited participants, everything proceeds in good order. But watch out when the proper balance is disturbed!

The *LDL cholesterol,* which is produced by the liver and constitutes the majority of the total cholesterol number, contributes to many essential cholesterol-related operations, such as the production of adrenal gland hormones. But LDL also has the potential to become too numerous in the blood, with the excess LDL molecules playing a central role in the process of atherosclerosis, or hardening of the arteries. That's why LDL cholesterol is often referred to as "bad" cholesterol.

Triglycerides are also blood fats, which, though not the same as cholesterol, are close cousins. Like LDL cholesterol, triglycerides can contribute to coronary artery disease when they become too numerous.

HDL cholesterol—which is made in the liver, intestines, and other parts of the body—is known as "good" cholesterol because it operates in the blood as a kind of security force that removes unruly, excess LDL molecules. (The HDL particles have the help of a protein, ApoE. For more on this, see Chapter 3 of *Controlling Cholesterol.*)

A note on triglycerides: Recent research indicates that triglycerides—the "other" blood fats that are usually tested at the same time you have your cholesterol blood test—present more of a danger than we had previously thought.

Triglycerides—which come into the body through the diet as large lipoproteins called *chylomicrons,* or are manufactured in the liver and elsewhere in the body from energy sources such as fat and carbohydrates—have long been suspects in the cholesterol "murder mystery." But until recently, there wasn't enough evidence to indict. Now considerable blame for cardiovascular disease lies at the feet of this lipid. In particular, a Harvard study published in *JAMA* on September 18, 1996 (pp. 882–88), concluded that triglyceride levels in the blood "appear to be a strong and independent predictor of future risk" of heart attack—especially when the total cholesterol of the person was elevated.

So now that we have our three main party participants, we need some transportation to get them around the circulatory system—and once again the liver has responded, with a kind of "stretch limo" known as *very low-density lipoprotein (VLDL).*

The VLDL particles move the LDL, triglycerides, and assorted other blood fats and proteins out into the far reaches of the arteries and blood vessels. The HDL cholesterol appears to move about on its own, policing the bloodstream and participating in the removal of excess, out-of-control LDL molecules.

In healthy blood, a cholesterol "party" can proceed without danger or damage. Unfortunately, however, the majority of us have a circulatory system that harbors cholesterol concentrations that require some sort of external "police intervention"—such as a low-fat diet, functional foods, or statin drugs—to restore order.

One problem is that the liver may produce too many potentially dangerous LDL cholesterol guests—far more than the body can handle.

Another possible problem is improper functioning of LDL "receptors" in the liver and on cells throughout the body. These are supposed to enforce a kind of "curfew" by pulling in the LDL for constructive duties in the body's cells when it's time to end their tour of the bloodstream.

A third potential difficulty is that the HDL cholesterol "security force" may be smaller than average and thus unable to handle a normal-size contingent of the LDL cholesterol. Or the HDL force may be of normal size, but the LDL molecules may be so numerous that they overwhelm the ability of the HDL to rein them in. According to prevailing theory, HDL molecules help "mop up" or remove the excess LDL from the bloodstream.

Finally, *free radicals*—or unstable oxygen molecules—are present in varying degrees throughout the body. These are true "party crashers," troublemakers who are poised to attack loose LDL cholesterol molecules, oxidize them (much as oxygen causes iron to rust or food to go rancid), and thus begin the process of atherosclerosis.

Now here's a brief scenario to show you how a cholesterol "party" can go totally out of control:

Too much LDL cholesterol spills out of the VLDL "stretch limo" and begins to float unrestrained throughout the bloodstream. The sheer numbers are too much for the HDL security force to handle.

Soon free radicals attack and oxidize the loose LDL molecules, which then become bloated, stick to vessel walls, and contribute to the buildup of plaque. Plaque is a yellowish swelling on the inside wall (intima) of a blood vessel, which tends to become *calcified,* or covered with deposits of calcium. Excessive triglycerides may add to this destructive process.

Over time the arteries become harder, as plaque accumulates and causes the vessel to become more narrowed *(occluded)*. Finally, the blood flow may be shut off entirely. If this happens with a coronary artery, which feeds blood and oxygen to the heart tissue, a heart attack results. If the blockage occurs with an artery leading to the brain, a thrombotic stroke may strike.

Clearly, this sort of "wild cholesterol party" must be brought under control immediately—before too much excess LDL cholesterol or triglycerides get out into the bloodstream. And the first step in protecting yourself is to learn how to evaluate your cholesterol risk.

Evaluating Your Risk: What Is Your Cholesterol Starting Point?

First, if you haven't done so already, you'll need to schedule a blood test that will provide you with your main cholesterol measurements. In particular, you must know these numbers:

- Total cholesterol;

- "Bad" LDL (low-density lipoprotein) cholesterol;

- "Good" HDL (high-density lipoprotein) cholesterol;

- Ratio of total cholesterol to HDL cholesterol; and

- Triglycerides.

Note: Most blood labs now include the ratio automatically, but if yours doesn't, it's easy to calculate. Just divide the total cholesterol number by the HDL cholesterol number.

The charts on pages 30 and 31 give you your blood-fat risk profile at a glance—including the two main blood fats (or *lipids*), cholesterol, and triglycerides.

To help you read them accurately, here are a few bits of basic information about each chart. Chart 1, which is the main one highlighted throughout this book, focuses on your risk if you are an adult age 20 or older *without* any personal history of heart or vessel disease.

Chart 2 is for adults age 20 or older *with* a personal history of such disease. As you can see, if you've been diagnosed with clogging of the arteries, or if you've had a prior heart attack or thrombotic stroke (involving a blood clot), the requirements are more stringent for keeping your lipid levels low.

Chart 3 is for children and teenagers, ages 2 to 19. Because they are still developing physically, their risk values differ from those for adults. In general, however, their lipids should be lower than those for an adult without cardiovascular disease.

You'll note, by the way, that certain risk categories in the adult chart—such as the "low" risk category and certain values for HDL cholesterol—are not included for children. The reason is that not enough scientific data is available for children for me to include these particular items in the chart.

As you read the chart, keep in mind these fundamental facts about cholesterol risk:

- **Low total cholesterol is desirable.**
Reason: Most of it is made up of "bad" LDL cholesterol—which may become oxidized and contribute to the buildup of plaque in the vessels.

- **Low LDL cholesterol is desirable.**
Reason: Excess LDL is vulnerable to oxidation by free radicals and the buildup of plaque.

- **High HDL cholesterol is desirable.**
Reason: High "good" HDL cholesterol is associated with a lower risk of cardiovascular disease and the ability of the body to remove excess LDL molecules.

• A low ratio of total to HDL cholesterol is desirable.

Reason: The higher your proportion of HDL cholesterol in relation to total cholesterol, the more HDL you'll have at your disposal to remove excess "bad" LDL molecules. Remember: The greatest component of total cholesterol is LDL cholesterol.

• Low triglycerides are desirable.

Reason: Like cholesterol, they can contribute to the development of blockages in the coronary arteries leading to the heart. But, in addition, they tend to lower the HDL cholesterol and make the LDL cholesterol more *atherogenic* (more likely to contribute to plaque deposits). They may also signal other diseases, such as diabetes mellitus, and they may cause pancreatitis.

Now, here are some further explanations of the columns and rows in the charts:

The first column, entitled "risk level," refers to the level of cardiovascular risk—including vessel disease, heart attacks, and strokes—in which your different cholesterol and triglyceride readings could place you. Obviously, it's best to have measurements that put you in the "low" category for all cholesterol components. But an "acceptable" classification is all right too.

On the other hand, if you find that you are in the "borderline" category for any type of blood fat, you should strive—through the Compound Effect and functional food strategies described later in this book—to lower your risk. A "high" risk result in any category places you at high risk for atherosclerosis, the "hardening of the arteries" that involves buildup of plaque in the blood vessels and an increased likelihood of a heart attack or stroke.

The "total cholesterol" column refers to the total amount of cholesterol that is circulating in your bloodstream.

As you know, total cholesterol includes many different subcomponents—most predominantly, the "bad" LDL cholesterol which is indicated in the third column.

The subcomponent of total cholesterol included in the fourth column of the chart is "good" HDL cholesterol.

In the fifth column, you'll see a reference to "total/HDL ratio," or the ratio of total cholesterol to "good" HDL cholesterol. I've included this measurement because many cholesterol researchers regard it as the most important figure in evaluating cardiovascular risk from cholesterol.

To get this ratio, you simply divide the total cholesterol by the HDL cholesterol. So if your total cholesterol is 200 mg/dl and your HDL is 50, you would divide 200 by 50 to get a ratio of 4.0. This would place you in the "acceptable" category if you are a man without heart or vessel disease but in the "borderline" category if you are a woman without such disease.

Finally, the sixth column provides risk ranges for the other important blood fat (lipid) that is circulating in your bloodstream: triglycerides.

Because of the increasing awareness, over the last ten years, of the serious cardiovascular risk posed by triglycerides, let me say still another word about them and their position in the chart—and our authority for setting certain levels of risk.

The Harvard study in the September 18, 1996, issue of *JAMA,* which I cited earlier, focused on the triglyceride levels of nearly 15,000 men in the Physicians' Health Study. The researchers found that participants who suffered heart attacks had median levels of triglycerides of 168, as compared with 132 for those who didn't suffer an attack.

As a result of such studies, my current recommendations, which are reflected in the accompanying charts, can be summarized this way:

• Patients *without* a history of heart or vessel disease should have triglyceride levels no higher than 150, and if possible below 125.

• Those *with* a history of heart or vessel disease should have triglyceride readings below 125.

How can you lower your triglycerides?

Some of the best natural, nondrug techniques involve losing weight; eating fish that are high in omega-3 fatty acids (like salmon, halibut, and sardines); and exercise, which tends to "burn off" the excess triglycerides in the blood.

Ironically, eating a healthy high-carbohydrate diet, which leans heavily toward fruits and vegetables, may actually raise triglyceride levels. But balancing such a diet with moderate exercise should keep triglycerides within a safe range for most people.

Finally, you can see that the risk values for men and women in the charts are often different, especially in the columns for "HDL cholesterol" and "total/HDL ratio." In particular, men tend on average to have lower HDL cholesterol and higher ratios than women. The main reason for this variation can be traced to the natural differences in the way male and female bodies produce blood lipids and organize their physiological systems to protect against cardiovascular disease.

A note on blood-fat measurements: The measurement used in this chart for cholesterol and other lipids (or fats) is *milligrams per deciliter,* or *mg/dl.* In your blood test results, all the values

CHART 1:

Your Blood-Fat Risk in a Nutshell

Adults Ages 20 and Older *Without* Personal History
of Heart or Vessel Disease

Risk Level	Total Cholesterol	LDL Cholesterol	HDL Cholesterol	Total/HDL Ratio	Triglyc-erides
Low	<180 mg/dl	<120	M: >55 F: >65	M: <3.5 F: <2.5	<125
Acceptable	180–199	120–129	M: 46–55 F: 56–65	M: 3.5–4.2 F: 2.5–3.0	125–150
Borderline	200–240	130–160	M: 35–45 F: 40–55	M: 4.3–5.5 F: 3.1–4.2	151–200
High	>240	>160	M: <35 F: <40	M: >5.5 F: >4.2	>200

All values in milligrams per deciliter (mg/dl)
M = male / F = female / < = less than / > = greater than

should also be in milligrams per deciliter (mg/dl).
But if your lab uses milli*moles* per liter (mmol/L),
as is sometimes the case in European countries,
you can convert to mg/dl by multiplying the
mmol/L figure by 38.7.

What's the Best Blood-Fat Predictor?

What's the best predictor of cardiovascular disease on a
cholesterol blood test?

There is an increasing tendency to place a heavy
emphasis on LDL cholesterol as the key component to
watch—especially for people who have a history of heart

CHART 2:

Your Blood-Fat Risk in a Nutshell

Adults Ages 20 and Older *With* Personal History
of Heart or Vessel Disease

Risk Level	Total Cholesterol	LDL Cholesterol	HDL Cholesterol	Total/HDL Ratio	Triglyc-erides
Acceptable	<160 mg/dl	<100	M: >45 F: >55	M: <2.5 F: <2.5	<125
Borderline	160–200	100–120	M: 35–45 F: 40–55	M: 2.5–4.0 F: 2.5–3.5	125–200
High	>200	>120	M: <35 F: <40	M: >4.0 F: >3.5	>200

All values in milligrams per deciliter (mg/dl)
M = male / F = female / < = less than / > = greater than

CHART 3:

Blood-Fat Risk for Children, Ages 2–19

Risk Level	Total Cholesterol	LDL Cholesterol	HDL Cholesterol	Triglyc-erides
Acceptable	<170 mg/dl	<110	NR	<125
Borderline	170–200	110–130	NR	125–200
High	>200	>130	<35	>200

All values in milligrams per deciliter (mg/dl)
M = male / F = female / < = less than / > = greater than /
NR = no recommendations

Total/HDL ratios for children and teenagers have been
omitted because of a lack of research on HDL and ratios for
these age groups

disease. In any event, it's essential for cardiac patients to get that LDL measurement below 100, as the chart indicates.

But there is also strong evidence suggesting that the ratio of total cholesterol to "good" HDL cholesterol may be the best of all the cholesterol tests in predicting future cardiovascular disease.

Researchers from the Montreal General Hospital and McGill University in Montreal reported in *JAMA* in 1995 on a 12-year study of 3,698 men and women, aged 35 to 74. They discovered that the ratio provided as accurate a screening device as other current American cholesterol screening guidelines. (See *JAMA*, vol. 274, no. 10, Sept. 13, 1995, pp. 801–806.)

Those people who have genetically low HDL levels shouldn't despair! The trick is to accept the genetic problem you've inherited and work to offset it by focusing on other lipid subcomponents.

Suppose, for instance, that you are a 60-year-old woman with naturally low HDL levels—say, in the range of 35 or so. HDL is usually responsive to aerobic exercise. But no matter how long or far you run or swim, your readings remain the same, at about 35. Your total cholesterol stands at 190, a level that would in most cases be regarded as quite healthy. But because of your low HDL, your ratio is a decidedly unhealthy 5.4 (190/35, or 190 divided by 35, or 5.4).

What can you do? If you can't raise your "good" HDL total cholesterol, you should concentrate on lowering your total cholesterol—and the new functional foods may be your best bet in achieving this goal.

Let's assume that your diet is already relatively low in fat. Your daily intake of fat calories amounts to only about 26 percent of your total daily calorie intake. Also, your intake of saturated fats and *trans fats* (those that are hydrogenated or partially hydrogenated)—which pose a great danger in raising blood cholesterol levels—is only 8 percent of your total calories.

You could always try to cut your saturated-fat and trans-fat levels down still further, but if you do, you're afraid you wouldn't enjoy your meals as much.

So you turn to a cholesterol-lowering functional food, which contains a plant stanol ester extract. After being on the product for several weeks, your total cholesterol drops to 148. This gives you a ratio of 4.2—still not the ideal, but much healthier and in a lower cardiovascular risk category than the original ratio.

A Distant Cousin of Cholesterol: Homocysteine

Some experts believe that another component of the blood, called *homocysteine,* may eventually turn out to be an even better predictor of cardiovascular disease than cholesterol.

In fact, I've discovered in my own practice that for *some* people—who have special cardiovascular risk profiles—homocysteine does indeed seem to be a more important predictor of cardiovascular problems than cholesterol.

What is homocysteine?

Unlike cholesterol and triglycerides, it's not in the blood fat family. Rather, homocysteine is a product of the breakdown of the amino acid methionine in the blood. Amino acids, as you probably know, are often called the "building blocks" of protein. Scientists currently estimate that high levels of homocysteine are involved in up to 15 percent of all heart attacks and up to 40 percent of strokes.

From a close reading of the scientific literature, I've come up with this homocysteine cardiovascular risk profile:

Very high risk: 19 micromoles per liter or higher
High risk: 13–18 micromoles per liter
Moderate risk: 10–12 micromoles per liter
Low risk: 6–9 micromoles per liter
Very low risk: 5 micromoles per liter or lower

If you find yourself in the "moderate risk" category or higher, what can you do?

The treatment is simple: Begin to take a minimum of 400 micrograms (mcg) of folic acid per day, and preferably 800 micrograms. In addition, you should take 50 milligrams (mg) per day of vitamin B_6 and 400 to 500 micrograms (mcg) of vitamin B_{12}. Both the folic acid and the B_6 help bring homocysteine down. The B_{12} protects you against the risk of pernicious anemia. (High doses of folic acid can mask the development of pernicious anemia, which is characterized by a deficiency of vitamin B_{12}.)

These supplements cost relatively little and can be purchased in almost any pharmacy or supermarket. The results, moreover, can be dramatic.

My wife, Millie, dropped from a "very high risk" homocysteine score of 21 to a low risk status with a measurement of 7.6. She achieved this result by taking 800 mcg per day of folic acid, in addition to 50 mg per day of vitamin B_6 and 400 mcg per day of vitamin B_{12}. Another patient dropped from a moderately high homocysteine level of 12 down to the low category with a 6.

The examples from my own practice are abundant, but I think you get the point. So have your homocysteine level tested, and if it's high, go on folic acid, vitamin B_6, and vitamin B_{12}.

Note: Physicians have long realized that 400 to 800 mcg of folic acid should be taken each day by all women of childbearing age to lower the risk of neural tube defects and congenital abnormalities in their newborn children. In fact, the federal government has taken steps to fortify a number of foods with folic acid. Some popular cereals, such as Total, include enough folic acid in one serving to meet the daily requirement of 400 mcg.

In the last couple of years, this advice about taking extra amounts of folic acid has been extended from women of childbearing age to everyone concerned about preventing cardiovascular disease.

Unfortunately, most physicians don't test routinely for homocysteine levels at this time. You usually have to ask for the test, which is relatively expensive, and typically you have to wait several weeks for your blood to be sent to a distant lab for testing.

But I would recommend that you ask your doctor about this procedure and plug it into your regular medical exam routine. New technology, such as that now available at our Cooper Clinic laboratory, has enabled us to perform this test in just a few hours, and the cost has dropped by two-thirds.

Now that you have a good idea about where you stand in terms of your blood fat risk, you're in a better position to take action. And the first important step is to focus on what I call the "twin pillars" of natural cholesterol control—diet and exercise.

3

The Twin Pillars of Diet
and Exercise

For most people, the starting point for controlling cholesterol the natural way must be *diet plus exercise*—a traditional, well-established strategy, but one with a number of new features that were not apparent a decade ago.

To begin with, even I—as one of the world's most ardent advocates of fitness and healthy eating—have been surprised by the raw power that can be generated to lower cholesterol through traditional nondrug techniques.

Perhaps the best evidence that a lifestyle approach can work entirely by itself is the 1990 investigation conducted by Dr. Dean Ornish and colleagues from the University of California San Francisco School of Medicine. (See *Lancet,* July 21, 1990, pp. 129–33.)

The article describing their investigation—which was entitled appropriately "Can Lifestyle Changes Reverse Coronary Heart Disease?"—revealed that diet, exercise, and other "lifestyle" strategies *alone* can actually bring about a *reversal* of severe coronary atherosclerosis, or hardening of the arteries—without the use of lipid-lowering drugs!

Specifically, they put a group of patients on a regimen that involved a low-fat vegetarian diet, no smoking, stress-management training, and moderate exercise. As a result, their coronary artery blockages decreased. Overall, 82 percent of the patients who underwent the lifestyle treatments experienced improvement of their coronary artery disease.

The women in the study enjoyed a reversing of their disease after making only moderate lifestyle changes. All were postmenopausal, and none was on estrogen replacement therapy.

When this study was conducted, cholesterol-lowering functional foods weren't available, and our understanding about lowering cholesterol through the dietary use of soluble fiber, such as that found in psyllium and oats, was in its infancy. With these functional foods as a featured part of the program, the study results might have been even more dramatic.

In any event, it is clear that for many people, lifestyle strategies—such as a low-fat diet, a moderate exercise regimen, a stress-reduction program, and a functional food plan—are all that's required for treatment or prevention of coronary artery disease. Now let's look at the first "pillar" of a wise natural strategy: your diet.

The First Pillar: A Low-Fat Diet

The cornerstone for lowering your cholesterol and cardiovascular risk—as well as for weight control, reducing the risk of cancer, and various other benefits—is the low-fat diet.

How much can you expect to lower your cholesterol through diet alone?

I've discovered that most people who pursue a reasonably disciplined low-fat diet can reduce their total cholesterol by about 50 mg/dl. One patient of mine cut his measurements by 25 points simply by eliminating all cheese from his diet.

Of course, if you are able to stick to a relatively strict diet—such as the 20 percent fat diet I mention on page 40—you might lower your total cholesterol by much more. (Most of the reduction, by the way, will come from your "bad" LDL cholesterol—though those on a low-fat diet also often lose some of their "good" HDL cholesterol as well.)

What should a well-designed low-fat diet look like?

The best place to start is the Step I and Step II diets, which are the standard models suggested by the National Cholesterol Education Program (NCEP). Also, the American Heart Association recommends these diets—and I use them as a good, simple starting point for my own patients.

The Step I diet is the first one that people usually try because it's the less demanding of the two. If the Step I regimen doesn't lower cholesterol enough, the patient usually goes on to the more stringent Step II diet—and later may even move to still more rigorous eating regimens.

Here are the basic components of these two diets:

Step I Diet

● The calories you eat from *all fats* each day should constitute 30 percent or less of your total calorie intake. So if you typically consume 2,500 calories of food per day, no more than 750 of those calories should come from fats.

● *Saturated fats,* such as the fats found in butter and whole-milk products, should comprise 8 to 10 percent or less of your total calories for the day. So if you are on the above 2,500-calories-per day routine, your saturated-fat calories should be no higher than the 200-to-250 calorie range.

● *Polyunsaturated fat,* which is present in such foods as corn oil, may amount to as much as 10 percent of your total calories.

● *Monounsaturated fat,* which is found in relatively large quantities in olive oil and canola oil, may constitute as much as 15 percent of daily calories.

● You should eat fewer than 300 mg of *dietary cholesterol* per day.

● *Carbohydrates,* which are present in large amounts in vegetables and fruits, should constitute 55 percent of your daily calories.

● *Protein,* which is abundant in such foods as fish and animal meals, should constitute about 15 percent of daily calorie intake.

● The *total calories* you consume should be just enough to enable you to achieve and maintain a healthy weight—and that target weight should be determined in consultation with a physician or registered dietitian.

Step II Diet

● As with the Step I diet, the calories you eat from *fat* each day should constitute 30 percent or less of your total calorie intake.

● But here's a difference: *Saturated fat* intake should represent less than 7 percent of your total daily calories, instead of the 8 to 10 percent recommended for Step I.

● *Polyunsaturated fat* may amount to as much as 10 percent of your total calories.

- *Monounsaturated fat* may constitute as much as 15 percent of your daily calories.

- Another difference: You should eat fewer than 200 mg of *dietary cholesterol* per day.

- *Carbohydrates,* which are present in large amounts in vegetables and fruits, should constitute 55 percent of your daily calories.

- *Protein,* which is abundant in such foods as fish and animal meals, should make up about 15 percent of daily calorie intake.

- Like the Step I diet, the *total calories* you consume should amount to just enough to enable you to achieve and maintain a healthy weight—and that target weight should be determined in consultation with a physician or registered dietitian.

Because the restriction on fats, and especially saturated fats, is so important, I sometimes recommend that before my patients give up on dietary control, they should try even lower amounts of fat intake than those suggested by the NCEP diets. This, in turn, means that the percentage of carbohydrates (but not protein) will go up.

For example, taking in 20 to 25 percent of total calories as fat may work for some people. Or it may be helpful to cut intake of saturated fats well below the 7 percent mark—say, to the 5-to-6 percent range, or even lower.

With a 20 percent fat diet, the final dietary calories would be divided this way: 65 percent carbohydrate, 15 percent protein, and 20 percent fat. The fats, in turn, might be divided so that about 10 percent are monounsaturated, 5 percent polyunsaturated, and 5 percent saturated.

A Trans-Fats Update

As you design your diet, remember that it's particularly important to reduce the amount of *trans fats* in your diet.

During the past decade, there has been increasing emphasis on the dangers posed by these hardened fats, which occur when polyunsaturated fats from vegetable oil are combined with hydrogen atoms through the process of hydrogenation. Indicated on food labels through such terms as *hydrogenated* or *partially hydrogenated,* trans fats can be found in relative abundance in such foods as stick margarine and commercial crackers and cookies.

A 1997 report from the Harvard School of Public Health Nurse Study, published in the *New England Journal of Medicine* (vol. 337, pp. 1491–99), revealed some startling new facts about the threat of trans fats. In evaluating more than 80,000 women, 34 to 59 years of age, the researchers found that trans fats posed even more of a cardiovascular risk than saturated fats.

Specifically, the investigators concluded that if an individual cut her intake of trans fats by only 2 percent, she would reduce her risk of coronary disease by 53 percent! In contrast, lowering the consumption of saturated fat by 5 percent would reduce the risk of coronary disease by 42 percent. *In other words, cutting trans fats had more impact on coronary disease than cutting saturated fats.*

So it's essential, in designing your own cholesterol-lowering diet, that you reduce your intake of trans fats, as well as your consumption of saturated fats.

An Egg Exception?

One of the most surprising new findings since I wrote *Controlling Cholesterol* concerns the egg, which many physicians and dietitians have eliminated from their patients' cholesterol-control diets.

In the past, the perceived problem with eggs was that because they are very high in cholesterol, they tend to increase the dietary intake of this blood fat too much.

One medium-size egg contains about 213 mg of cholesterol, while a large hard-boiled egg with shell removed has more than 270 mg. This would appear to pose a big problem for those on the Step II diet described above, because the maximum amount of cholesterol allowed per day is less than 200 mg.

But a 1999 study from the Harvard School of Public Health found that one egg per day had no substantial impact on the risk of stroke or coronary heart disease among the nearly 38,000 men and more than 80,000 women who were followed over a 14-year period. (See *JAMA,* vol. 281, April 21, 1999, pp. 13878–94.)

The one exception to the good news was that the study's diabetic participants had more coronary heart disease associated with higher consumption of eggs than did the non-diabetic participants.

The researchers speculated that the reason that healthy people showed no adverse cardiovascular reaction to eggs was that the negative impact might be offset by protective nutrients in the eggs—such as antioxidants, folate (a member of the B-vitamin family), other B vitamins, and unsaturated fats. (Eggs are relatively high in monounsaturated fat.) Also, they said that the eggs might have helped raise the levels of "good" HDL cholesterol.

The investigators concluded that heart-healthy diets should focus mostly on reducing the intake of saturated fat and trans fat, rather than on limiting total fat or dietary cholesterol.

My own feeling about this study is to assume a temporary wait-and-see posture before you add eggs to your diet. We simply need more information before we can justify a drastic change in diets—especially for those at high risk for cardiovascular disease.

Also, this particular study was based on questionnaires, and the responses in such a survey are generally less reliable than those involving a more controlled look at the participants' habits. In addition, the researchers apparently conducted no regular monitoring of blood-lipid levels, and so we can't really know what effect the eggs were having on blood cholesterol.

On the other hand, I have no objection to allowing up to one egg per day, even for those with mildly elevated cholesterol—but with these provisos:

Aside from your slightly high total or LDL cholesterol, you should otherwise be at relatively low risk—with no personal history of heart disease and no other major coronary risk factors, such as high blood pressure. Also, if you begin to consume up to one egg per day, you should undergo a blood test after about a month, just to see what the impact is on your total and LDL cholesterol.

If there isn't an increase in your total or LDL cholesterol, then you may be safe in your new dietary adventure—and I'd say continue with your consumption of eggs in small amounts.

But if your experience conforms to previous studies on eggs and cholesterol, you'll probably find that your total cholesterol increases on average by 4 percent—or 8 points for a person with total cholesterol of 200. That may not seem like much, but remember: An increase of only 1 percent in your total cholesterol translates over time into a 3 percent increase in your risk of getting coronary heart disease! An egg a day hardly seems worth the risk.

The Second Pillar: Exercise

Any complete program for controlling cholesterol should include regular aerobic (endurance) exercise—but again, I've changed my exercise prescription somewhat over the last decade. So what remains the same—and what has changed?

Here is an overview of some of the most important shifts that have influenced me in recent years.

What's the Same?

I have no doubt that exercise is still necessary for elevating the "good" HDL cholesterol in most people.

We've known for a long time that exercise—especially aerobic or endurance exercise done over a sustained period of 20 to 30 minutes or so at least three days per week—can raise the level of "good" HDL cholesterol by 5 to 10 percent or more. That fact remains as true today as it was ten years ago.

Another fact that we have known for a while is that exercise can lower levels of blood triglycerides, which have been linked to a higher cardiovascular risk.

More recently, however, we've developed a better understanding of how this works. The mechanism seems to involve the release during exercise of an enzyme known as *lipoprotein lipase,* or LPL, which breaks down the triglycerides for use as body fuel. (See *Science,* May 30, 1997, p. 1325.)

What's Changed?

A major shift is in our understanding of *how hard you must work* to derive significant cholesterol benefits from exercise.

We used to assume that a vigorous workout was

required to raise "good" HDL cholesterol to adequate levels. And it is certainly true that you must keep up a minimal level of intensity while working out to get the full cholesterol-balancing effect, according to a 1996 report in the *American Journal of Epidemiology* (vol. 143, no. 6, pp. 562–69).

Still, the level of exertion tends to be well within the capability of most people of every age. In the above study, for instance, to experience an elevation of "good" HDL cholesterol, it was necessary to walk or jog at the relatively undemanding rate of at least about 14 minutes and 30 seconds per mile. Somewhat more effort—a pace of about 11 minutes per mile—was required to trigger decreases in total cholesterol, "bad" LDL cholesterol, and triglycerides.

Another study expressed the way to cardiovascular benefits in terms of total distance. The researchers said that the most significant improvements in your HDL levels will tend to occur if you jog approximately 7 to 14 miles per week. (See *Archives of Internal Medicine,* Feb. 27, 1995, pp. 415–20.) Jogging only 7 miles per week translates into just 1 mile a day—or a little over 2 miles per day, three days per week.

We also have learned that *moderate exercise can benefit HDL levels in the elderly.*

Light workouts by elderly Japanese men and women, averaging about 75 years of age, resulted in significant increases in "good" HDL cholesterol, according to a 1995 study from Fukuoka University in Nanakuma, Japan. (See *European Journal of Applied Physiology,* vol. 70, 1995, pp. 126–31.) The men and women in the study worked out at low intensity on a treadmill for 30 minutes per session, three to six times per week, over a nine-month period.

Does it take months to achieve these HDL benefits? Not at all. Other studies have shown that *only one ses-*

sion of exercise on a stationary bicycle at low intensity—at a relatively low 50 percent of maximal aerobic capacity—can produce beneficial changes in blood lipids shortly after the exercise.

In one of these studies, triglycerides were 18 percent lower, and "good" HDL cholesterol rose by 8 to 9 percent. Also, both total and "bad" LDL cholesterol fell by 4 percent immediately after the exercise session. (See *Journal of Applied Physiology,* vol. 79, July 1995, pp. 279–86.)

The HDL Cholesterol of Men Versus Women

Is there a difference in the way the blood lipids of men and women respond to exercise?

Some studies have shown that the HDL levels of men benefit more from exercise than those of women. But as we'll see in chapter 9, a report in the *New England Journal of Medicine* (May 16, 1996, pp. 1298–303) revealed that substantial increases in HDL cholesterol occurred in serious female runners as they increased their running distances.

Another group consisting of women averaging 62 years of age walked an average of about 55 minutes per day, five days per week for six months, at a low intensity of 54 percent of their maximum heart rate. At the end of the six-month period, they experienced significant declines in the total cholesterol, triglycerides, and ratio of total to HDL cholesterol. (See *Canadian Journal of Cardiology,* vol. 11, Nov. 1995, pp. 905–12.)

From all indications, there is every reason to treat men and women equally as far as exercise and HDL cholesterol are concerned—even if we were inclined not to do so in the past.

But whether you are male or female, what should you do in *practical* terms to enjoy maximum HDL protection?

A Simple But Powerful Exercise Program

Not everyone's HDL cholesterol responds to exercise. I have a number of patients who have low HDL cholesterol, but no matter how much they work out—up to and including marathon training—they can't budge those HDL measurements by one milligram per deciliter.

On the other hand, *most* people *can* benefit from a few low-intensity workouts every week, such as a vigorous walk or bike ride. So if you are currently pursuing regular endurance or aerobic activity, stay with it.

If you are sedentary, you should immediately begin a program to maximize your HDL protection. Here's a suggested sequence of steps to get started rather painlessly:

- *Get a medical exam first.* If you haven't been working out, you want to be absolutely sure that you don't have hidden heart problems or other health concerns.

- Set aside three days per week, with a day of rest in between. On those days—say, Monday, Wednesday, and Friday—allot 20 minutes for a vigorous walk. Walk as fast as you can, but keep the pace comfortable. You're in this for the long haul, and after you've continued for a month or more, you'll experience significant increases in your endurance and leg strength.

- After two to three weeks, increase your walking time to 25 to 30 minutes. Continue at this pace for another three weeks.

- After six or eight weeks of this regular activity, add an extra day to your routine, with the same time and pace you're using on the other days.

• Using this graduated technique, work up
during the next few months to an hour per
session at higher rates of walking speed.
You can keep track of how fast you're
going by measuring your distance with a car
odometer and then keeping a record of the
minutes that it takes you to cover a given
distance.

After this, it's up to you. You will have begun to enjoy significant HDL benefits *after your very first workout.* Now
you're in the process of developing a higher level of fitness—which our studies at the Cooper Institute and elsewhere have shown will decrease your risk of dying from
heart problems and all other causes. (See *JAMA,* Nov. 3,
1989, pp. 2395–401.)

Furthermore, you're in a position to put your exercise
together with your diet to benefit from what might be
called a *diet-exercise synergy.*

The Diet-Exercise Synergy

Diet and exercise don't just operate independently—they
can actually work together to lower your cholesterol.

A positive interaction between diet and exercise in
lowering "bad" LDL cholesterol emerged in a July 2,
1998, report in the *New England Journal of Medicine*
(vol. 339, pp. 12–20).

The researchers, from Stanford University School of
Medicine, found that during a one-year period, men and
women who followed the more restrictive, low-fat NCEP
Step II diet *and also engaged in aerobic exercise* were
able to lower their LDL levels by 15 to 20 points on average. In contrast, those who didn't exercise failed to lower
their LDL levels to this extent. The researchers concluded that it's quite important to include aerobic exercise

with a diet for maximum reduction of "bad" LDL cholesterol.

But the benefits of the diet-exercise combination don't stop here. Many studies have shown that these two strategies, operating both alone and together, can produce still another benefit for your blood lipids: a reduction in obesity and percentage of body fat.

The Body-Fat Connection

Obesity has been getting bad press in recent years because it has been identified as an important risk factor for high blood pressure, heart disease, adult-onset diabetes, and different types of cancer.

Obesity is also a major concern as you take steps to control your cholesterol. For one thing, adding to your percent of body fat will often result in a reduction of your levels of "good" HDL cholesterol. (See *Circulation,* Nov. 4, 1997, pp. 3248–50.)

Being obese will also raise your levels of total cholesterol, "bad" LDL cholesterol, and triglycerides. (See *International Journal of Obesity,* vol. 20, 1996, pp. 1081–88; *JAMA,* July 8, 1998, pp. 140–46.)

There's an additional concern about *where* your fat accumulates. Increases in *subcutaneous fat* on the trunk of the body—such as just under the skin around the abdomen—may have a negative effect by lowering your levels of "good" HDL cholesterol.

Also, those with a high waist-to-hip ratio (found by measuring and comparing the circumferences of those two parts of the trunk) tend to have more of a small, dense form of "bad" LDL cholesterol. This topic is covered in chapter 10, as one of the "next steps in cholesterol control."

So what's your healthy level of body fat?

The desired body-fat range for men is 19 percent of total body weight or lower, and for women it is 22 percent or lower. For the most accurate measurements, you should go to a clinic that does skin fold measurements with calipers or, even better, underwater hydrostatic weighing. But what if you don't have access to such a clinic?

How to Calculate Your Body Fat

There is a rough measurement you can use without equipment to find the general body-weight levels that will be likely to limit you to a healthy level of body fat. With this method, which is my personal variation on what is known in exercise physiology as the Mahoney Formula, the calculation is slightly different for women and men.

Note: When you do your calculations, you will come up with two numbers, which represent a range of body weight. This range corresponds to a healthy range of body fat. Therefore, if your real weight falls within the range of these numbers, your body fat will fall within the healthy range. (These formulas are derived from studies of normal adult body types. Growing adolescents, highly conditioned competitive athletes, and others with a high proportion of bone or muscle mass may actually have a low percentage of body fat, even though they are relatively heavy.)

The Formula for Women

To find a body weight containing the healthy range of 18 to 22 percent body fat:

Step One: Determine your height in inches.

Step Two: Multiply the number in Step One by 3.5.

Step Three: Subtract 108 from the result in Step Three. This number represents your approximate weight for 18 percent body fat—or the *lower* weight in pounds for a healthy range.

Step Four: Now, multiply the result in Step Three by 10 percent (0.10).

Step Five: Add the result in Step Four to the result in Step Three. This will give you a body weight that corresponds with about 22 percent body fat—or the *upper* end of the acceptable range for you.

Here's how this formula would work if you are a woman who is five feet three inches in height: First, you find your height in inches, which would be 63 inches. Then, you multiply that by 3.5 to get 220.5. Next, you subtract 108 from 220.5 to get 112.5—or the number of pounds that represents about 18 percent body fat for you.

Now, you multiply 112.5 times 0.10, a calculation that gives you 11.25. Finally, add 11.25 to 112.5, and you'll get approximately 124 pounds—or the upper range of body weight that represents about 22 percent body fat.

So your desired body weight range for a healthy percent of body fat (18 to 22 percent) is 112.5 to 124 pounds.

What if your actual weight is *above* 124, or 22 percent body fat? You probably need to lose weight. Consult your physician.

What if your actual weight is *below* 112.5, or 18 percent body fat? That's most likely all right—and may be expected if you are particularly athletic or have a naturally low-fat body type.

But generally, for optimum health, a woman's body-fat percentage should be above about 12 percent of total body weight—for several reasons. Women, even more than men, must guard against losing too much body fat. For one thing, premenopausal women who are too thin may upset their hormonal balance by producing too little estrogen—and as a result experience amenorrhea, or the loss of at least three periods in a row.

Second, a woman with too little body fat will be at a higher risk for osteoporosis, or thinning of the bones, which leads to spontaneous fractures.

Also, a rapid weight loss may indicate another serious health problem, such as gastrointestinal problems or cancer.

Finally, excessively low weight may signal an eating disorder.

The Formula for Men

To find a body weight containing the healthy range of 15 to 19 percent body fat:

Step One: Determine your height in inches.
Step Two: Multiply the result in Step One by 4.
Step Three: Subtract 128 from the result in Step Two. This is your approximate weight for 15 percent body fat—or the *lower* weight in pounds for a healthy range.
Step Four: Multiply the result in Step Three by 10 percent (0.10).
Step Five: Add the result in Step Four to the result in Step Three. This will give you a body weight that corresponds to about 19 percent body fat—or the *upper* end of the acceptable range for you.

So if you're a man who is five feet ten, your height in inches is 70. Multiply that by 4 to get 280. Then subtract

128, and you'll end up with 152 pounds, or the weight that will give you 15 percent body fat.

Now multiply 152 by 10 percent (0.10), and you'll get 15.2. Add that to 152 pounds, and you'll have 167.2 pounds as the upper range of healthy body weight for you—a figure that includes about 19 percent body fat.

In contrast to women, there is less concern for men whose body fat dips below the 15-to-19 percent range—especially those men who are competitive athletes. On the other hand, an unusual or rapid weight loss—or weight loss accompanied by a decline in muscle mass—can suggest health problems that should be evaluated by a physician.

Another Alternative: The BMI

Some physicians and physiologists prefer a measurement known as the *body mass index,* or BMI. To obtain your BMI, divide your body weight in kilograms by your height in meters squared. Or multiply your body weight in pounds by 705 and divide by your height in inches squared. A score of less than 25 is acceptable; from 25 to 30 is overweight; and above 30 is obese.

I usually avoid using the BMI to estimate body fat or obesity because I believe it doesn't adequately take into account those who may weigh much more than average due to heavy bone structure or musculature.

Many times, for instance, I've examined professional football players whose BMI would suggest that they are hopelessly overweight and obese. But a more precise measurement has in many cases revealed that they have only 5 or 6 percent body fat. (The ideal range for an adult male is in the range of 15 to 19 percent.) The reason for this disparity, of course, is that these athletes are naturally heavy-boned, and they spend a lot of time in the weight room working out. (The body-fat formulas I suggested at the beginning of this section do a somewhat better job of taking into account bone and lean body mass.)

With this introduction to the traditional "twin pillars" of natural cholesterol control, you're prepared to move beyond the traditional to one of the most amazing medical strategies that has ever come to my attention as a preventive medicine specialist.

4

The Breakthrough Discovery of Functional Foods

As I was walking through the large double doors of the Cooper Clinic recently, I sensed that I was also moving through a gateway into a new era of medical treatment—an amazing drugless world that would have transcended even my wildest dreams a few years before.

A flight of fancy? Not at all!

With growing excitement, I realized that what I was feeling so deeply was rooted in the firmest scientific reality. Indeed, I was crossing the threshold of a new age of functional foods that can lower the risk of heart and vessel disease dramatically by controlling cholesterol naturally—with no medications and no side effects.

Yet to understand where we are, it helps to understand how we got to this momentous juncture in medical history.

So let's take a quick trip through time to see how a series of seemingly unrelated events brought us to the new way of life we are about to enjoy:

Circa 3000 B.C.: Chinese peasants find that the seeds of a wild legume are edible and can even be used for medicinal purposes. The soybean eventually becomes a high-protein staple of many human and animal diets.

Circa 2500 B.C.: An Indian farmer discovers that the seeds and seed husks of a common oatlike plant can be ground up and used to make nutritious bread products. Psyllium soon becomes a common component of diets in this part of the world.

A.D. 1862: A German scientist discovers a molecule in peas that is later identified as a *plant sterol* or *phytosterol*—a carbon-based chemical compound.

1980s and early 1990s: Pine trees begin to fall throughout Finland as scientists discover that the "tall oil" contained in wood pulp contains relatively high amounts of *plant stanols,* or a fully saturated form of plant sterols.

What do these events have in common?

Taken together, they have paved the way for the advent of this new era of nutriceuticals, or specially designed functional foods, that can actually control cholesterol—the natural way.

The products are proliferating even as you read these pages, so it's hard to keep track of exactly what is available on your supermarket shelves. Even as I've engaged in some research related to functional foods, I've become increasingly aware of how fast this field is moving—and how much potential the scientific findings have for me as a physician, and for you as a patient. But here is a partial listing of products that can help improve your cardiovascular health without drugs:

- **Benecol**—margarinelike spreads, salad dressings, and yogurt produced by McNeil Consumer Healthcare, a unit of Johnson & Johnson.

  Operative cholesterol-lowering ingredient: plant stanols, derived from the "tall oil" wood pulp of pine trees.

- **Take Control**—a margarinelike spread produced by the Lipton division of the Dutch conglomerate Unilever.

  Operative ingredient: plant sterols, derived from soybeans.

- **Phytrol**—a food additive developed by Forbes Medi-Tech, a biotechnology company based in Vancouver, British Columbia, and produced and distributed by Novartis Consumer Health SA, a division of Novartis, a health-care and nutrition conglomerate based in Basel, Switzerland. Possible products containing the additive include margarine, salad dressings, and mayonnaise.

  Operative ingredient: Plant sterols (phytosterols), extracted from wood pulp.

- **Psyllium**—a grain-seed husk included in various Kellogg Company products, such as its Bran Buds cereal. Psyllium and other related cholesterol-lowering products, such as oats, are produced through Kellogg's Ensemble Functional Foods Company.

  Operative ingredient: a potent natural soluble fiber from the husk of the psyllium seed, a grain commonly grown in India.

To understand how these agricultural and scientific breakthroughs evolved, let's look back at some of the discoveries that occurred in the last century. The logical place to begin is with what I call a "tall oil tale."

A "Tall Oil Tale"

Fifty years ago, as a Finnish logger who might be called Pekka felled pine trees in the dark forests of his frigid homeland, he assumed that the raw wood products he provided would be used for sauna linings, home building, newsprint, and paper manufacture.

He could hardly have suspected that a life-saving elixir might be hiding in the vast conifer timberland, which covered more than three-fourths of his nation. Nor could he have known that the ingredients for this elixir lay before him, in the fatty components hidden in the common wood pulp of his tall pine trees—components known as "tall oil" because they come from the towering trees.

Yet even as Pekka wielded his ax and saw on the edge of the arctic circle, scientists were starting to connect molecules in pine trees with blockages that were developing in Pekka's own blood vessels, slowly shutting off the flow of blood and oxygen to his heart.

Of course, the logger wasn't aware that he was developing deadly atherosclerosis. He also had no idea that in the early 1970s, scientists would confirm that he was a citizen of a nation that had the world's highest cardiovascular-related mortality. Yet the very wood pulp Pekka was producing would begin in the 1990s to play a decisive role in lowering cardiovascular risk in Finland. Food products manufactured from the "tall oil" in the pulp would cause cholesterol levels to plummet by up to 16 percent in some villages in the northland. Cardiovascular risk and disease—including the health threat Pekka himself faced—would decline accordingly.

But when Pekka was cutting down trees at mid-century, neither researchers nor practicing physicians yet understood what a broad-based threat that out-of-control cholesterol represented. More information was required before they could comprehend the importance of the plant products as an antidote in the form of a kind of "anticholesterol." In a sense, the discovery of the antidote had preceded the diagnosis of the problem.

The Discovery of "Anticholesterol"

The process of discovery began in Germany in 1862, when researcher G.M.R. Beneke published a study saying he had found a kind of "cholesterol" in peas.

Beneke's conclusion was reasonable, given the history of research in this area. A series of studies during the eighteenth century had gradually unveiled the chemical nature of cholesterol as a component of gallstones and liver bile. Finally, in the early nineteenth century, the French chemist Michel Chevreul gave the flaky white substance a name: *cholesterine.*

Scientists determined, in later experiments through the nineteenth century, that cholesterol was present in blood, brain tissue, chicken eggs, and other unlikely places. So it was natural for Beneke to assume that he had found one more spot where cholesterol "resided"—the common pea.

But he was wrong.

What he had actually discovered was a molecule that *looked* much like cholesterol. Later studies showed that it even *acted* like cholesterol in humans and animals. But what looks and acts like a duck isn't always a duck.

In fact, as scientists learned a few decades later, Beneke had stumbled upon a *plant sterol,* or *phytosterol,* which, like cholesterol, is made up of a combination of carbon and alcohol atoms. Yet the biological impact of different types of phytosterols is the exact opposite of cholesterol.

As we know now, cholesterol—especially "bad" LDL cholesterol—is a major factor causing the buildup of deadly plaque and blockages in the arteries. But phytosterols can have the opposite effect, as a kind of "anticholesterol." They have the power to enter the body, push aside the cholesterol, and save your arteries from destruction.

In the nineteenth century, of course, no one had any inkling about any of this—least of all Beneke, who thought all along he was probably dealing with cholesterol. But science abhors uncertainty and error, and by the turn of the twentieth century, other researchers had corrected his mistake and embarked on studies to determine exactly what this mysterious phytosterol was all about.

Because much of the research fell into the category of pure science at this point—without any reference to possible benefits for human health—the progress was slow. There was just no pressure at the time to find a miracle cure for the greatest killer-disease in Western society.

Still, the work went on. In 1929 R. Schönheimer— conducting pure research without knowing the future implications of his work—published another report in Germany to the effect that plant sterols did not absorb well into the bloodstream of rabbits.

About twenty years later, research by D. W. Peterson, which was published in 1951 in the *Proceedings of the Society of Experimental Biology and Medicine,* established a connection between the intake of phytosterols and reduced blood cholesterol. Specifically, he discovered that a particular kind of plant sterols, *sitosterols,* which were extracted from soybeans, could lower cholesterol levels in chickens. A year later, a researcher from Delaware, O. J. Pollak, succeeded in using plant sterols to prevent the development of high cholesterol (hypercholesterolemia) in rabbits.

It was only a short step from these animal experiments for Pollak to move on to human subjects—and to conduct a landmark study that would become perhaps the most important event in introducing cholesterol-lowering nutriceuticals to the world.

The New Era Dawns

In research published in the journal *Circulation* in 1952, Pollak recruited 26 adult participants, whose initial blood tests revealed total cholesterol levels ranging from 126 to 414 mg/dl. Their average measurement was 256, or in the "high" risk level indicated on the cholesterol risk charts on pages 30 and 31. (However, it's important not to project our current knowledge in a critical way back into the minds of researchers in the early 1950s. Even into the 1980s, many clinics and physicians believed that total cholesterol levels as high as 300 or even 350 were quite normal.)

By today's standards, the typical participant in Pollak's study was at very high risk for developing hardening of the arteries (or atherosclerosis) and a heart attack. Did Pollak understand this, or was he simply driven by the opportunity to lower cholesterol as a purely academic challenge?

We really don't know. Most likely it was the latter. Without realizing the extent to which his studies would one day benefit millions, Pollak took the next step—to go beyond the experiments with chickens and rabbits and to find an effective response for human beings.

The key ingredient that he tested in his experiment wasn't too appetizing. He wanted his volunteers to eat rather large quantities of a certain crude powder every day for two weeks. The physical properties of the powder—a plant extract containing a form of plant sterol, *sitosterol,* which is a natural component of vegetable oils and fats—were rather forbidding, to say the least. And Pollak pulled no punches in his description of the substance in a 1953 medical journal article.

He said that sitosterol "has a low specific gravity, is light, bulky and lumpy. It has a chalky appearance and taste, a dirty, off-white color, and a gritty, sticky consistency." (See *Circulation,* vol. 7, 1953, pp. 702–703.)

Not exactly the kind of snack you'd choose to put out for dinner guests! In fact, I wonder how he managed to hold on to the participants, who were given 5 to 7 grams of the "dirty, gritty, sticky" powder every single day.

But they stuck with the program—and helped Pollak compile some rather incredible evidence about the effect of the plant sterol extract on blood cholesterol. He reported that after the two-week period, the sitosterol powder had reduced the "mean average" cholesterol of the participants from the starting level of 256 to 173.5 mg/dl. (See *Pharmacological Therapy,* vol. 31, 1985, pp. 177–208.)

When he broke his subjects into groups with different cholesterol levels, he calculated these further results:

- a decline of 12.6 percent for those whose cholesterol was below 240;

- a drop of 22 percent for those with cholesterol above 240; and

- an amazing plunge of 39 percent for those whose total cholesterol was above 285.

Pollak also discovered another important feature of sitosterol. He kept his subjects off the plant extract for two to three weeks, gave them another round of blood tests, and found that their cholesterol levels had risen right back up to the original readings. In other words, the seemingly magical plant-based antidote could lower cholesterol quickly, but it had no staying power or carryover effect. To enjoy any ongoing benefits, you had to stay on it regularly and indefinitely.

With what we know now about the dangers of cholesterol in the human bloodstream, if Pollak's findings had burst onto the research scene within the past decade instead of in the 1950s, scientists and practicing physicians alike would have started to cry, "The answer to heart disease!"

But Pollak was a man ahead of his time. Although other research followed, confirming and building upon Pollak's findings, his landmark study sat quietly on the shelves of lipid research for nearly three decades, awaiting other investigations that would place his work in its proper context. During this period, there was simply no pressure to push forward with treatment applications because we still didn't understand the true dangers of cholesterol.

From Sterols to Stanols

In 1977 three other scientists—M. Sugano, H. Morioka, and I. Ikeda—took up the cause. They found what appeared to be an even more potent plant extract—a *plant stanol*—which is a completely saturated form of a plant sterol. In experiments with rats, which these three researchers published in the *Journal of Nutrition*, they concluded that *sitostanol*, which is a type of plant *stanol*, could be even more effective than the plant *sterol* that Pollak had used (vol. 107, pp. 2011–19).

In 1981 researcher Ikeda, who had participated in the above experiment, confirmed with another team of scientists that sitostanol could also lower blood cholesterol in rabbits. (See *Journal of Nutrition Science and Vitaminology,* vol. 27, 1981, pp. 243–51.)

Breakthrough Discoveries

After the alarming nature of the danger posed by cholesterol was recognized, the first line of defense chosen by practicing physicians was what has come to be called "lifestyle" changes—including a low-fat, low-cholesterol diet and regular endurance exercise.

But with many patients, these preventive measures weren't enough, and so physicians prescribed cholesterol-controlling drugs. Finally, during the 1980s, the stage was set for the ultimate step forward in the functional food movement. The early research by Pollak and other groundbreaking scientists had laid the foundation. Practicing physicians and the general public understood the danger. All that remained was to come up with a product that tasted good—and lowered cholesterol significantly.

The Birth of Benecol

Scientists in Finland, led by Tatu A. Miettinen of Helsinki University, perhaps the world's premier researcher into the impact of plant stanols on cholesterol, began to push food producers to come up with a solution to the problem of "gritty" plant sterols and stanols. Clearly, no one wants to chew on wood pulp. The trick was to find a way to combine the plant extract with real food products that had an acceptable taste. Dr. Ingmar Wester and other scientists at the Raisio Group in Finland responded with resounding success.

In 1989 Dr. Wester led his team at Raisio to develop a means of *fat esterification* for the plant stanol extract. This chemical process changes the unappetizing raw sitostanol into a fat-soluble *plant stanol ester,* which can then be included in margarine, salad dressings, yogurt, and other common food products.

Now research began to move along more rapidly. The first clinical study on the process was done in 1990, and five more clinical studies were conducted with fat-soluble stanol esters in the period between 1991 and 1995.

In 1992 Raisio also began a long-term clinical study, the North Karelia Stanol Study, in a rural Finnish province. Villagers were given a rapeseed (canola) margarine containing the plant stanol ester.

The study results were published in 1995 in the *New England Journal of Medicine*—and are described in more detail in chapter 6. But here's a quick summary: The scientists found that the margarine with the plant extract could lower total cholesterol by an average of more than 10 percent. Also, "bad" LDL cholesterol declined by an average of more than 14 percent. And those numbers just reflect the averages. Many people who have used these extracts for only two to three weeks find that their total and "bad" cholesterol levels decline by even greater percentages—as much as 22 percent or higher.

With such promising research, the plant extracts were soon taken out of the laboratory, manufactured for the general public as a rapeseed (canola) oil margarine, and sold in Finland under the brand name Benecol. And now Benecol is available in the United States as well.

The Soybean Scenario

You'll recall that some of the early animal experiments with cholesterol-lowering plant extracts focused on the ancient Chinese legume, the soybean. Unilever decided to take the soybean route in its research, with rather successful results.

In the late 1980s, Unilever scientists started exploring putting soybean extracts into foods. First they ascertained the safety of the ingredient when it was combined with other foods. Then they turned to possible nutriceutical benefits, including lowering cholesterol.

After reviewing several studies comparing the impact of plant *stanols* and plant *sterols* (saturated and unsaturated components of vegetable oils and fats), Unilever decided that the effects of each extract on cholesterol were substantially the same—and they chose to take the sterol route.

One key study—conducted by researchers from the Unilever Research Laboratorium in the Netherlands and published in 1998 in the *European Journal of Clinical Nutrition*—focused on 95 volunteers, averaging about 45 years of age, who had normal to slightly elevated total cholesterol levels. The participants were about equally divided between men and women.

The randomized, double-blind study was designed so that the subjects spent four periods of 3.5 weeks eating different types of margarine. (It was logical for Unilever, as the world's leading manufacturer of margarine and spreads, to select margarinelike products.) These included:

- a spread with soybean sterol extracts;

- one with rice-bran sterol extracts;

- one with shea-nut sterol extracts;

- Benecol margarine, containing plant stanol extracts; and

- a control margarine containing no special sterol or stanol nutriceutical ingredients.

The participants assigned to each group consumed daily amounts of margarine that were comparable to what they would have eaten apart from the study. Specifically, during each 3.5-week period, they consumed 30 grams of margarine per day, divided into two daily servings, at lunch and dinner. This would be the equivalent of a total daily intake of about one ounce, or three to four pats of a spread.

Researchers J. A. Weststrate and G. W. Meijer found that the rice-bran and shea-nut spreads had no effect on the participants' cholesterol. Neither did the control margarine.

But both the soybean-based sterol spread and the Benecol spread improved blood lipids in a similar way. Specifically, within only a 2.5-week period, each of these spreads lowered total cholesterol by an average of 8 percent, and "bad" LDL cholesterol by an average of 13 percent. Also, neither affected blood concentrations of "good" HDL cholesterol.

Weststrate and Meijer concluded that their findings confirmed previous studies done by Miettinen and his colleagues on the benefits of Benecol. But they also said that the spread containing sterol esters from soybean oil was just as effective as the Benecol. (See *European Journal of Clinical Nutrition,* vol. 52, 1998, pp. 334–43.)

As a result, Unilever chose not to put the sterols through the additional process that turned them into stanols. Instead, they developed a process using sterol esters derived from soybeans, and they produced the Take Control spread. (In Europe it's called "Flora pro-activ" or "Becel pro-activ.")

The Phytrol Additive

A small Vancouver-based biochemical firm, Forbes Medi-Tech, developed another food additive called *Phytrol.* This product, which can be added as a cholesterol-lowering agent to margarine or other foods, is based on a plant sterol from "tall oil" wood pulp—much like Benecol. But the Forbes approach is close to that of Unilever because the plant extract doesn't go through the process that turns the sterol into a stanol. Swiss-based Novartis has joined with Forbes to produce various cholesterol-lowering foods.

In a biochemical sense, as one Forbes scientist has put it, the Phytrol technique falls between the Benecol and Unilever processes. Yet if a series of preliminary studies is any indication, the food products that Novartis is making with the Phytrol additive may produce results similar to those of Benecol and Take Control.

Phytrol studies—which were first conducted successfully on animals and are now being done on human subjects—have shown significant reductions in blood cholesterol levels.

- According to an October 1996 report from Forbes, a trial was conducted with 12 adult men suffering from high blood lipids and cholesterol (hyperlipidemia). After taking 1.5 grams of the Forbes plant sterol extract daily for ten days, the subjects who were at highest cardiovascular risk experienced an average cholesterol reduction of 38 percent.

- In April 1996 a similar small study was done with patients having normal cholesterol levels. The result was a decrease in "bad" LDL cholesterol by as much as 17 percent in men and 10 percent in women.

Studies on the Phytrol additive are still being conducted, but from all indications, this additive seems to be on the same research track as Benecol and Take Control.

Designed Versus Traditional Functional Foods

With the increasing number of food products that are able to lower cholesterol, it's easy to lose track of which one does what. One way I keep my thinking organized in this new, exploding field is to distinguish between what I call *"designed" functional foods* and *"traditional" functional foods.*

Designed Functional Foods

With this category of nutriceuticals, scientists develop chemical processes to produce concentrated extracts or additives, which are able to lower cholesterol in ways that would be impossible for ordinary foods. Then the extracts are altered chemically so that they can be combined with ordinary foods. The result is a specially "designed" functional food. Though genuinely "natural," these products go through the additional chemical and manufacturing processes that give them their special power. These are produced by Johnson & Johnson, Unilever, and Novartis, which I've described in the preceding pages.

Traditional Functional Foods

A second approach to cholesterol-lowering products emphasizes what I would call *traditional functional foods.*

These are foods that have an inherent health or medicinal effect, without the need for additional extracts or chemical changes. In most cases, these foods have been cultivated and used by humans for centuries. But neither the growers nor the consumers had any idea until very recently about the powerful health effects that these products possessed.

The main traditional functional foods that have the ability to lower cholesterol are those that contain *soluble fiber*—including the psyllium-containing products from Kellogg. Fiber-containing foods have been available for millennia as a main staple of the diet in many lands. Also, farmers have suspected for a long time that certain medicinal benefits might be associated with some of the grains.

Now, with a rash of recent scientific studies, a movement has begun to market and encourage consumption of these "ancient" foods in the war against cholesterol. Currently, some of the prime candidates for cutting cholesterol can be found in the great grain family—including psyllium and oats.

The Soluble-Fiber Solution

Fiber—a carbohydrate substance that makes up much of the solid part of many fruits, vegetables, and grains—can be divided into two types: insoluble and soluble.

The best short definition distinguishing the two is that insoluble fiber *does not* dissolve in water or in the digestive tract. Soluble fiber, by contrast, *does* dissolve in these environments.

Foods containing significant amounts of *insoluble fiber*—such as wheat bran, corn bran, and "hard" or "crunchy" vegetables like broccoli—are often recommended to promote bowel regularity. Also, they may lower the risk of diseases of the colon, such as colon cancer and diverticulitis (inflammation of pouches on the colon).

Insoluble fiber has also been associated with a lower risk of heart disease—though some mechanism other than lowering of cholesterol seems to be involved. For example, insoluble fiber may improve the body's regulation of blood glucose and insulin. (See *American Journal of Preventive Medicine,* vol. 9, 1993, pp. 197–202.)

In contrast, *soluble-fiber* foods—such as oats, oat bran, psyllium, apples, beans, strawberries, and citrus fruits—have been linked directly to a lowering of blood cholesterol in humans. Specifically, if you consume at least 7 or 8 grams of soluble fiber per day, and preferably more, you can expect this functional food to lower your total cholesterol by 3 to 10 percent. The precise benefit will depend on the quantities you eat and the way your body's digestive and biochemical systems respond.

A number of scientific studies in the 1970s and early 1980s showed that various types of fiber—and especially soluble fiber—could lower cholesterol levels. The foods that researchers identified as having this nutriceutical power included apples, oat bran, soy hulls, guar gum, various beans and legumes, and pectin (a fiber found in apples and certain other fruits). (See George V. Vahouny and David Kritchevsky, eds., *Dietary Fiber: Basic and Clinical Aspects,* New York: Plenum Press, 1986, p. 310.)

Even during this early period, I strongly advocated that my patients with high cholesterol eat muffins, pancakes, and other foods that were made from oat bran. It was apparent to me that a patient might well benefit from this functional food—and, with other dietary adjustments, might be able to lower or even eliminate a drug requirement.

In a surprise finding during this initial exploration into soluble fiber, scientists reporting in the *Archives of Internal Medicine* in 1988 discovered that a common laxative, Metamucil (psyllium mucilloid), which was made from the ancient Indian grain psyllium, also had strong cholesterol-lowering properties.

These researchers, who studied the effect of this psyllium derivative on 26 men, found that, on average, the subjects who took 3.4 grams of psyllium per day for eight weeks had nearly a 15 percent drop in their total cholesterol. They also experienced a 20 percent decrease in their "bad" LDL cholesterol.

The biological mechanism, they speculated, was the ability of psyllium, which contains significant amounts of soluble fiber, to bind cholesterol in the intestine and prevent the reabsorption of the cholesterol into the bloodstream through the intestinal walls (vol. 148, p. 292).

As the concern about high levels of cholesterol increased, scientists and manufacturers accelerated the drive to find just how effective grains and other soluble-fiber foods are in lowering cholesterol. Here are some recent research results on psyllium, in particular:

- A Kellogg Company study of more than 400 adults, published in 1997 in the *Journal of Nutrition,* revealed that adults who had high cholesterol but ate a psyllium-enriched cereal as part of a low-fat diet, could improve their lipid profiles over what they could achieve on a low-fat diet alone. Specifically, the researchers found that those eating the psyllium cereal had 5 percent lower total cholesterol and 9 percent lower "bad" LDL cholesterol (Oct., vol. 127, pp. 1973–80).

- Fifty-one men and women eating a diet consisting of 15 grams per day of soluble dietary fiber for eight weeks—including psyllium, pectin, guar gum, and locust bean gum—experienced reductions in average total and "bad" LDL cholesterol of 6.4 percent and 10.5 percent respectively. (See *American Journal of Cardiology,* vol. 79, Jan. 1, 1997, pp. 34–37.) Their "good" HDL cholesterol and triglyceride levels remained unchanged.

- In a 1994 Australian study, 81 men, who averaged 50 years of age and had mildly elevated levels of total cholesterol, ate a soluble-fiber cereal for six weeks. The soluble fiber was 86 percent psyllium and 14 percent oatmeal and barley. The participants experienced an average decline of 3.2 percent in their total cholesterol and 4.4 percent in their "bad" LDL cholesterol. (See *Medical Journal of Australia,* vol. 161, Dec. 5–19, 1994, pp. 660–64.)

Don't Forget Your Oats!

In tandem with this recent emphasis on psyllium, scientists have continued investigating the effects of oat bran and other fibers on cholesterol. We have known for a number of years that the soluble fiber in these oats can have a significant effect in lowering total and "bad" LDL cholesterol levels. More recently, investigators have discovered a number of other interesting and useful facts:

● A diet high in *oat bran*—consisting of an average daily intake of 9 grams of soluble fiber from oat bran—resulted in a 24 percent reduction in the ratio of "bad" LDL cholesterol to "good" HDL cholesterol. (See *Journal of the American Dietetic Association,* vol. 96, December 1996, pp. 1254–61.)

● A small daily intake of soluble fiber from *oats*—2 to 10 grams per day—produced a small but significant decline in total and "bad" LDL cholesterol, according to a 1999 Harvard School of Public Health report. (See *American Journal of Clinical Nutrition,* vol. 69, January 1999, pp. 30–42.)

In this analysis of 67 scientific trials, the researchers found that only 3 grams of soluble fiber from oats (from 3 servings of oatmeal, 28 grams of cereal per serving) could produce a decrease of 5 mg/dl in both total and "bad" LDL cholesterol. On a cholesterol level of 200, this would amount to a decline of 2.5 percent.

● *Full-fat rice bran*—which contains minimal soluble fiber but a great deal of lipid-lowering rice-bran oil—can lower cholesterol almost as effectively as oat bran in humans with high cholesterol levels, according to a 1998 study from the Department of Medicine, University of California, Davis Medical Center, Sacramento. (See *Journal of Nutrition,* vol. 128, May 1998, pp. 865–69.)

This six-week investigation involved one group on a placebo, a second group on 84 grams per day of full-fat rice-bran product, and a third group on 84 grams per day of an oat-bran product. In the rice-bran group, total cholesterol decreased by 8.3 percent and "bad" LDL cholesterol dropped by 13.7 percent. With the oat bran, the improvement was even more dramatic: a 13 percent drop in total cholesterol and a 17.1 percent decrease in "bad" LDL cholesterol. The researchers found no consistent effect on "good" HDL cholesterol or on triglycerides.

● Ground *fresh rhubarb stalks*—consisting of 66 percent insoluble fiber and 8 percent soluble fiber—succeeded in lowering cholesterol levels significantly in a four-week 1997 study of ten Canadian men with high cholesterol. (See *Journal of American College of Nutrition,* vol. 16, December 1997, pp. 600–604.)

The participating men ate 27 grams per day of ground rhubarb-stalk fiber—an amount that would have included just under 3 grams per day of soluble fiber. Yet even with this minimal amount, they experienced on average an 8 percent lowering of total cholesterol and a 9 percent decline in "bad" LDL cholesterol.

The researchers, who were from the Department of Agricultural, Food, and Nutritional Science, University of Alberta in Edmonton, concluded that rhubarb-stalk fiber is effective in lowering serum (blood) cholesterol concentrations—especially "bad" LDL cholesterol—in hypercholesterolemic men (those with high blood cholesterol). Also, they noted that the use of rhubarb crops is under-utilized for this functional food purpose.

A Quick Biology Lesson

A major factor that makes *designed* functional foods different from the *traditional* category is that traditional fiber-based foods operate through a different biological mechanism than that of plant-extract foods.

Here's a summary of how designed and traditional functional foods operate in their own special ways to lower your cholesterol.

Mechanism 1: Designed Functional Foods

As you know, we use the term *designed* for functional foods like Benecol and Take Control because they are a combination of regular table foods *plus* scientifically developed extracts. The extracts in these products include concentrated versions of regular plant stanols or sterols, which pack a huge wallop in their ability to affect human cholesterol levels.

How exactly do the plant stanol and sterol extracts lower cholesterol levels?

The answer lies well beyond the range of the naked

human eye, far down at the molecular level. Plant stanols and sterols closely resemble cholesterol molecules. In fact, they are so similar to cholesterol that they have the power to compete successfully with cholesterol for absorption through the wall of the small intestines and into the bloodstream.

In the typical human body, a total of about 1,400 mg of cholesterol enter the intestine each day. Of these, 400 mg come from food in the diet, and the liver produces the other 1,000 mg as a component of the yellowish bile fluid.

Once this cholesterol arrives in the small intestine, it is absorbed for the first time (in the case of dietary cholesterol) or reabsorbed (in the case of cholesterol from the liver) through the intestine walls. This process occurs with the help of *micelles,* which are tiny droplets of fat.

In effect, these micelles act as molecular "carts" or "vehicles" that transport the cholesterol into the body and bloodstream. Without a ticket on the micelle carts, cholesterol can't get through the intestinal wall. Instead it's washed out of the body as waste in bowel movements.

The function of the plant stanols (or sterols) is to "kick out" cholesterol from the micelles so that it can't enter the bloodstream. Plant sterols and stanols can do this because they are identical to cholesterol in molecular structure, yet somehow they possess an "aggressive streak" that enables them to prevail over the cholesterol. So if enough of the plant stanols can be placed in the small intestines, as much as 80 percent of those 1,400 mg of cholesterol that enter the intestine every day can be eliminated.

This operation, which can be triggered by a designed functional food like Benecol, is highly effective. But it's also quite different from what happens with a traditional functional food containing soluble fiber, such as oats or psyllium.

Mechanism 2: Traditional Functional Foods

How does soluble fiber work to lower cholesterol?

Most scientists feel that psyllium, oats, oat bran, rhubarb, and similar foods, which contain soluble fiber, operate by "binding" or "tying up" the bile that comes into the intestine from the liver—and causing it to be excreted from the body.

The bile contains most of the cholesterol that gets into the body through the intestine wall. So the more soluble fiber that enters the intestine and ties up the bile, the less cholesterol will enter the bloodstream—and cause a buildup of plaque in the vessel walls.

Recent research has fine-tuned this explanation as far as psyllium is concerned. Chemical alteration of the synthesis of bile acid appears to be the mechanism by which psyllium lowers "bad" LDL cholesterol, according to an August 1992 study in the *Journal of Lipid Research* (vol. 33, pp. 1183–92).

In that investigation, 26 men, averaging 44 years of age, consumed 15 grams per day for 40 days of either psyllium or a placebo. The psyllium lowered "bad" LDL cholesterol significantly in many of the participants. Furthermore, its operation was associated with an increase in *bile acid synthesis*—or chemical changes in the bile acid in the intestines—in those whose "bad" LDL levels dropped by more than 10 percent. (Bile acid is the *emulsifer*—or agent controlling suspension of one liquid in another—that assists with fat and cholesterol absorption.)

The important thing to note here is not the scientific details of the biological operations of designed versus traditional functional foods. Rather, you should simply focus on how different each process is: The *designed* foods "kick out" the cholesterol from the micelles, while the *traditional* foods attack cholesterol through the bile. It's apparent that each mechanism operates independently—and so to maximize the cholesterol-lowering action, both types of food should be incorporated in your diet.

> **Note:** There is also a third class of biological mechanisms that occur with different cholesterol drugs. These vary depending on the medication prescribed. The *statin drugs,* for instance, operate by interfering with the synthesis of cholesterol in the liver, while the *bile acid sequestrants* have their main impact on the bile that enters the intestines. We'll go into the chemical and biological work of these medications in more detail in chapter 6. For now, just keep in mind that drugs offer one more way to pile up an additional cholesterol-lowering effect in your body.

With this introduction to the main types of functional foods and their biological operations, you're now ready to take the next step. It's time to develop your own individual functional food strategy—by learning to control your cholesterol naturally but powerfully through the Compound Effect.

5

The Functional Food Strategy: Capitalizing on the Compound Effect

The functional food strategy I'm advocating in these pages is ready-made to help those who keep putting off medical exams, neglecting low-fat diets, and making excuses that they simply don't have time for regular exercise.

This revolutionary new approach to lowering cholesterol and cardiovascular risk typically sets into motion a chain of health-enhancing events that sometimes seem almost impossible to stop once they are started. At least that was the experience of Scott, a high-powered executive in his late forties who had never put his health on the front burner.

How Scott Finally Saved His Own Life

For years Scott had postponed having a complete medical exam, including a blood test, because he felt he just couldn't fit an appointment into his busy schedule. His career had been exploding, with promotion after promotion and with stock options contributing to a hefty investment portfolio.

But now, as he approached 50, Scott gave in to his wife's insistence that he pay better attention to his health. He was overweight and sedentary, and his energy levels had been flagging in recent months. She worried that with his poor fitness level and family history of heart disease, she might wake up one day to find that he wasn't going to be around to enjoy his worldly accomplishments and bulging stock holdings.

As it happened, Scott took this first step toward better health in the nick of time. The doctor who evaluated him discovered that in addition to being 15 pounds overweight and having a father who had died of a heart attack in his early fifties, Scott was suffering from mildly elevated blood pressure. Also, an exercise stress test revealed that in terms of cardiovascular fitness or aerobic endurance, he was in very poor condition.

As if his dismal showing on these cardiovascular risk factors weren't enough, the blood test showed that his cholesterol was seriously out of control.

His total cholesterol was 262 mg/dl, or well up into the "high" risk category. (See chart 1 on page 30.) His "bad" LDL cholesterol was also in the "high" risk range at 181.

There was some good news, in that his "good" HDL cholesterol was in the "acceptable" category at 53. His triglycerides were also in the "acceptable" range at 143.

But with his results, his ratio of total cholesterol to HDL cholesterol ended up in the middle of the "borderline" risk category at 4.94.

Overall, then, Scott's cholesterol, when combined with his other cardiovascular risk factors, made him a likely candidate to suffer from premature heart or vessel disease or a stroke. His doctor recommended strongly that he begin a preventive program immediately, with a three-month trial period devoted to lifestyle adjustments, such as a low-fat diet, moderate endurance exercise, and weight loss. If the nondrug treatments succeeded in lowering his blood pressure and cholesterol, he might be able to avoid medications. Otherwise there would be no other option but drugs.

But Scott felt immobilized because he had been down this route before. He knew he had to do something, and he really did want to avoid medications. But he also was afraid that he would fail with diet and exercise now, just as he had done before.

Then his doctor referred him to a colleague of mine. Together they designed a start-up program that featured *only* designed cholesterol-lowering functional foods containing the Benecol plant stanol ester. Scott took in enough of the Benecol spreads and salad dressings each day to enable him to consume at least 3 grams daily of the operative plant stanol ester.

After only two weeks of eating the Benecol—which required no effort or disruptive dietary changes on his part—Scott's lipid profile improved significantly. The numbers speak for themselves:

- His total cholesterol dropped to 242, a decline of 7.6 percent.

- His "bad" LDL declined to 156, a decrease of 13.8 percent—and a new, lower "borderline" risk classification.

- His "good" HDL rose rather unexpectedly to 58.

- His ratio of total to HDL cholesterol dropped to 4.17—which placed him in the "acceptable" range for this measurement, probably for the first time in his life.

- His triglycerides stayed about the same at 146.

His doctor assured him that if he responded like other patients, these numbers would improve still further as he continued to use the nutriceutical.

Scott was so encouraged that he decided to add an additional, very easy step in his emerging functional food strategy for the next two weeks: He included some traditional soluble-fiber products in his dietary program. These included psyllium cereals and oat-bran muffins, which enabled him to consume at least 10 grams of cholesterol-lowering soluble fiber per day.

With these extra dietary adjustments—which required only a little extra effort to buy and absolutely no sacrifice on his part because he liked the foods—Scott witnessed another drop in his cholesterol readings. A second blood test two weeks later showed these changes:

- His total cholesterol went down by another 10 percent, to 217—or well within the "borderline" category and approaching the "acceptable" threshold that begins below 200.

- His "bad" LDL cholesterol also dropped by 10 percent, to 140.

- His "good" HDL cholesterol stayed the same, at 58.

- His ratio of total to HDL cholesterol declined once again, this time to 3.74. This was far enough down in the "acceptable" to bring him within striking distance of the "low" risk category, which begins below 3.5.

- His triglycerides held steady in the same general range, at 141.

With such positive results at his four-week evaluation, we could see what I call the *Compound Effect* beginning to operate in Scott's body. I'll explain this effect in more detail below, but here's a preliminary definition:

The Compound Effect refers to the augmentation of one cholesterol-lowering technique, which operates through one biological mechanism, with another technique, which works through a different mechanism. The result is a multiple effect in controlling your blood fats.

In Scott's case, he used functional foods having two separate biological mechanisms—the designed plant stanol products and the traditional soluble-fiber items. Together these put Scott within striking distance of an "acceptable" range in all his cholesterol measurements.

But just as important, Scott was now *motivated.* He had witnessed dramatic changes in his blood fats, and he could see that much more would be possible—both with his cholesterol and also with his blood pressure. All that was required was for him to make some simple adjustments in his diet and physical activity—and stick to them!

Up to this point in his new program, Scott had made no attempt to lower the fat in his diet, embark on even a very low-demand exercise regimen, or lose weight. Yet now, in contrast to his half-hearted attitude in the past, he was actually eager to start changing his dietary and exercise habits.

If I were a betting man, I would have said it was a sure bet that he could bring his cholesterol numbers within at least the "acceptable" if not the "low" range. All he had to do was follow this simple plan that I have suggested to many other patients as well:

• Reduce your intake of fats below 30 percent of your daily calories (and your saturated fats below 10 percent);

- Lose that extra 15 pounds; and

- Begin to walk 20 to 30 minutes a day, three or four days per week.

Without the functional foods to get him started, Scott never would have had a chance, even with such a simple, undemanding plan. But this time he stuck with the program. By the end of the three-month trial period, he had brought all his blood fat numbers into the acceptable range and also lowered his blood pressure to a healthy level.

As Scott continues to cut fats out of his diet and increase the amount of his exercise, I expect that he will see even greater improvements in the future in his risk profile.

How to Bring the Compound Effect into Your Life

What can you learn from Scott's experience?

First of all, he was lucky enough to wake up to his health risks at just the right time—as functional foods for lowering cholesterol became available.

Second, he found that a functional food strategy wasn't something he had to spend hours or days formulating. In many ways, it was a no-brainer for a busy businessperson. All he had to do was substitute a tasty spread or salad dressing for the usual one he used—and good things began to happen in his body.

Third, as Scott saw good things begin to happen, the incentive intensified to do more. The functional foods had, in effect, provided him with the jump-start that he had lacked in the past in trying to stick to diet and exercise programs.

To bring the Compound Effect into your life as Scott

did, I'd suggest two simple steps—both of which he found to be important in increasing his motivation to lower his cholesterol.

First, identify a starting point or "baseline" against which you can measure your progress. This means that you should have a blood test before you begin, so you can watch your risk decline from test to test. I've discovered that there's nothing more affirming and inspiring for many people than to be able to see their cholesterol numbers decline in black and white.

Second, design a simple functional food strategy that incorporates several cholesterol-lowering nutriceuticals. This will serve as your personal action plan to help you bring your cholesterol numbers in line.

The Compound Effect: What It Is—And How You Can Use It to Control Your Cholesterol

The Compound Effect is a simple but potent principle in any effective cholesterol-lowering strategy—and has been enhanced immeasurably by the development of functional foods. Here's another capsule definition:

> *The Compound Effect refers to the increased power to lower or balance cholesterol that is achieved when you combine one approach to treatment with one or more separate approaches to treatment.*

The addition of extra treatments doesn't typically overlap with or substitute for the original treatment. Instead, through different biological mechanisms, the additional treatments increase the power of the overall treatment strategy.

For example, we've long known that a low-fat, low-cholesterol diet will lower total cholesterol and "bad" LDL cholesterol in most people. We've also been aware of the fact that endurance exercise will usually raise levels of "good" HDL cholesterol. More recently, we've learned that combining exercise with diet will actually make the diet work better in reducing cholesterol levels.

To take this one step further, we've known for several decades that if diet and exercise don't complete the job of controlling cholesterol, a cholesterol-lowering medication can be added to strengthen the treatment mix. In other words, the patient continues the diet and exercise but at the same time adds on a drug—and derives an augmented or *compounded* benefit.

The reason that multiple attacks on a cholesterol problem often work so well is that they frequently operate differently in the body. Going on a diet low in saturated fats, for instance, will lower circulating total and "bad" LDL cholesterol in the blood because saturated fat operates as a chemical trigger to produce more of these lipids in the blood.

During a one-year period, participants in a 1997 Northwest Lipid Research Clinic study reduced their "bad" LDL cholesterol levels significantly after cutting their intake of dietary fat. Specifically, they reduced their fat consumption from a range of 34 to 36 percent of total calories to a range of 22 to 28 percent. (See *JAMA,* Nov. 12, 1997, pp. 1509–15.) As a result, their LDL levels declined by about 5 to 13 percent, depending on the diet they used.

A separate dietary tactic—keeping intake of fat and cholesterol low—helps reduce cholesterol in the blood simply by a dietary subtraction process: Reducing your intake of fat and cholesterol means that your consumption of carbohydrates and protein will increase—if we assume your caloric intake remains the same. Consequently, your body has less fat and cholesterol to deal with on the inside.

A major advantage of introducing the Compound Effect into your life in the past was that if you were conscientious about making dietary and exercise changes, you might be able to reduce the dosage of cholesterol-lowering drugs—or avoid the necessity of medications altogether.

With the advent of the era of functional foods, this power of the Compound Effect to supplant the need for drugs can increase exponentially—as the experience of Adam demonstrates rather dramatically.

Adam's Amazing Luck

In his early forties, Adam had wrestled with high cholesterol for years. To make matters worse, his family history of cardiovascular disease portended a troubling future. His father had suffered a heart attack while still in his fifties, and an older brother was on cholesterol-lowering medications.

Despite the ever-present specter of what his loved ones had gone through, Adam couldn't seem to discipline himself to act wisely. His efforts to take care of his cholesterol problem by completely natural means—through a low-fat diet and aerobic exercise—failed.

For one thing, he just couldn't resist the pastries and other high-fat foods that tend to elevate total and "bad" LDL cholesterol. As a result, his daily intake of fat was close to 40 percent of his total daily calorie intake—when it should have been below 30 percent. Furthermore, as a result of those desserts, he was taking in far too much saturated fat—which made up more than 15 percent of his daily calories, when the figure should have been below 10 percent.

Also, Adam had neglected an endurance exercise program that a trainer had designed for him. He knew that the routine, which consisted of a combination of jogging and walking four days a week, had the potential to raise his "good" HDL cholesterol. But somehow other responsibilities were always cutting into his workout time, and he just couldn't seem to stick with the program.

Despite the failure of these nondrug remedies, Adam had resisted going on cholesterol-lowering drugs—for a couple of reasons. First of all, even though he knew the risk of side effects was minimal with the new statin type of medications, he didn't want to take any chances on possible liver problems, gastrointestinal disturbances, or the like. Also, he wanted to avoid any long-term commitment to drug therapy, which he knew would cost a considerable amount of money.

Yet Adam also knew that the clock was ticking on his cholesterol problem, and time was running out. A recent blood test had revealed that his total cholesterol was 274 mg/dl—which was well up in the "high" risk range, according to chart 1 on page 30. To put him at the "acceptable" level of risk, the reading should have been under 200.

His "bad" LDL cholesterol was 208. This number should have been below 130.

Adam's "good" HDL cholesterol—the subcomponent most strongly associated with protection against atherosclerosis—was only 34. This put him in the "high" risk category. His reading should have been above 45.

Also, Adam's triglycerides were somewhat elevated at 178. This reading should have been no higher than 150, or even better, under 125.

Finally, perhaps the most important cholesterol marker in predicting heart disease risk is the ratio of total cholesterol to "good" HDL cholesterol. An acceptable ratio for a man should be 4.2 or lower. But Adam's ratio stood at 8.1.

Just when Adam was on the verge of going along with his doctor's recommendations to begin medications, a stroke of good luck came his way. He was picked to participate in a study that had been designed to show the effect on human cholesterol of a wood-pulp-based extract—the plant stanol ester that I discussed in the previous chapter.

During the study, volunteers would either take a type of a margarinelike spread (in this case, Benecol), which contained the plant extract, or be assigned to a "control" group that took a spread without the plant extract. Adam enrolled in the eight-week study—and as it turned out, he was assigned to a group that received the active plant extract. He consumed one small pat of a margarinelike spread three times a day by putting it on his bread, vegetables, or other foods at each meal.

Adam followed the instructions faithfully—with dramatic results. After he had taken the product for only two weeks, his total cholesterol and "bad" LDL cholesterol began to decline significantly. By the end of the eight-week study, his cholesterol profile looked like this:

- Total cholesterol: 238 (down from 274)

- "Bad" LDL cholesterol: 184 (down from 208)

- "Good" HDL cholesterol: 41 (up from 34)

- Triglycerides: 91 (down from 178)

- Ratio of total cholesterol to HDL cholesterol: 5.8 (down from 8.1)

With these changes, Adam's cholesterol readings and cardiovascular risk profile improved significantly. According to the risk categories in the chart on page 30 his total cholesterol dropped from the "high" risk down into the "borderline" category. His triglycerides also declined into the "low" risk range.

Adam's "bad" LDL cholesterol was still in the "high" risk range. But unexpectedly, his HDL cholesterol actually went up, and his risk dropped from the "high" category down to "borderline."

Perhaps most important of all, his ratio of total cholesterol to HDL cholesterol came down dramatically from a spot far up in the "high" risk category, almost to the "borderline" level.

The Benecol margarine spread went a long way toward placing Adam in a position to balance his cholesterol *entirely* through natural meals. He is now ready to take full advantage of the Compound Effect.

Here is my specific recommendation about how Adam could employ a double-barreled, all-natural approach to his blood-lipid situation:

He should stick with the Benecol. But at the same time, he should reduce his daily intake of dietary fats below 30 percent of his total calorie intake. Adam's previous flirtations with such a low-fat diet had actually demonstrated that diet could make a difference in lowering his cholesterol—but he wasn't motivated.

In the past, Adam had proven too undisciplined to stay on an exercise regimen. But now, with a recent functional food success under his belt, he seemed to be more willing to try, and so an exercise program was now possible.

This enhanced sense of motivation is a common response. When someone sees how easy it is to lower cholesterol just by eating moderate daily amounts of a tasty margarine or salad dressing, the thought often comes to mind: "Maybe other dietary changes would work for me as well!"

What did a shift in diet mean in practical terms for Adam?

He settled upon a daily energy intake of 2,400 total calories, which he determined could satisfy his appetite and at the same time actually enable him to lose some weight. (A nutritional analysis showed that in the past, he had been taking in closer to 2,800 calories per day.) By losing weight, he was able to reduce his total and "bad" LDL cholesterol still further. (Various studies have shown that as your percent of body fat goes up, so does your cholesterol.)

As you can see, even a relatively limited application of the Compound Effect can make a huge difference in your cardiovascular risk.

Finding Your Personal Cholesterol Scenario

To understand how the Compound Effect can work in your own situation, it's helpful to think in terms of a comprehensive cholesterol-lowering strategy that involves one or more of three distinct *cholesterol scenarios*.

Each of these scenarios may feature some use of functional foods. But each also has the potential to lower or balance your cholesterol through biological mechanisms that the other scenarios lack. As a result, by taking advantage of more than one scenario, you will have access to multifaceted weapons that can fight your cholesterol battle in a variety of different ways.

The particular scenario or combination of scenarios that you and your physician choose will depend upon your special health needs and cholesterol profile. The three basic approaches include:

● **Scenario 1:** *The Lifestyle Scenario.*
This first approach emphasizes a low-fat, low-cholesterol diet; weight loss; and regular

endurance exercise. A limited reliance on functional foods may be appropriate here, but the keys are diet, weight loss, and exercise.

● **Scenario 2:** *The Functional Food Scenario.*
The second scenario features the cholesterol-lowering functional foods discussed in chapter 4. Lifestyle efforts, such as diet and exercise, are also essential if you hope to maximize the lipid-lowering effect. But functional foods are the cornerstone for this second approach.

● **Scenario 3:** *The Medication Scenario.*
If your cholesterol is still elevated or unbalanced after you move through the first two scenarios, you'll probably have to try a third technique—adding drugs prescribed by a physician. But even if you have to go on medications, in most cases, by relying on the first two scenarios, you will be able to lower your required dosage.

Here's a brief illustration of how the Compound Effect can work to improve your cholesterol profile as you move through each of these scenarios:

Assume that you are a 40-year-old woman who starts off with these lipid measurements: total cholesterol of 300; "bad" LDL cholesterol of 230; and "good" HDL cholesterol of 50. With these values, your ratio of total cholesterol can be calculated as 6.0.

From the cholesterol risk chart on page 30, you can see that you are in the "high" risk category for every one of these measurements except your HDLs—and you're "borderline" in that category. Also, you have a family history of heart disease, with both a mother and father who developed signs of atherosclerosis, or hardening of the arteries, before age 50.

Given your cholesterol profile, it's clear that you'll

have to make use of at least the first two scenarios, and perhaps the third as well.

Scenario 1

Through Scenario 1—involving a low-fat diet, weight loss, and endurance exercise—you should be able to lower your total cholesterol by 50 or 60 points, and most if not all of the reduction should come through a lowering of your "bad" LDL cholesterol. Also, the exercise should raise your HDL level by about 5 points. So now your total cholesterol should be down to about 240, your LDL cholesterol down to about 170, and your HDL up to 55.

Although you still need work on your blood lipids, your situation has improved considerably. Even though your LDL is still in the "high" range, your total cholesterol is now at the edge of the "borderline" category. Also, your HDL level is almost "acceptable," and your ratio is down to 4.36—or close to the "borderline" rating for women of 4.2.

In the past, a physician confronted with your situation might well have prescribed low-dose lipid-lowering drugs, such as one of the statins that we'll discuss in chapter 7. But today things have changed because you don't have to go directly to drug therapy.

Scenario 2

Instead, you can turn to Scenario 2—the new, intermediate cholesterol-lowering approach that features functional foods. Furthermore, by choosing different types of functional foods within this category, you can achieve a kind of mini–Compound Effect. Here's how this approach might work:

First, you could begin to use a designed functional

food like Benecol or Take Control. This would lower your total cholesterol by 11 percent through one type of biological mechanism. Then, you could up your daily intake of a traditional functional food, a soluble fiber such as psyllium or oats, and decrease your total cholesterol by about another 7 percent. This would occur through a separate biological operation in your body.

In numerical terms, the functional food would take your total cholesterol down to 214 from the 240 you achieved only through a low-fat diet. The soluble fiber would lower the measurement still more, by nearly 15 points to about 199. In other words, through completely natural means you have taken your total cholesterol from a very "high" risk level to an "acceptable" rating!

The other cholesterol values would also be in much healthier shape. You could expect your "bad" LDL to end up at about 129 ("acceptable"), and your ratio to be approximately 3.6—"borderline" for a woman, but much more desirable than the sky-high 6.0 that you started with.

Now reflect for a moment on what's happened here.

You have not only achieved a much more desirable cholesterol risk profile, but you have done it in systematic fashion by taking advantage of the step-by-step power of the Compound Effect. Furthermore, you have utilized only the first two cholesterol scenarios—and have not had to turn to the third scenario, which involves the use of drugs.

Each of the lipid-lowering mechanisms you used has operated independently, without any overlap. In other words, what you achieved through a low-fat diet was added on to the work of the Benecol. Then the impact of the soluble fiber was added to the reductions resulting from the first two techniques.

And let me reiterate: Unless an exercise stress test or

other diagnostic evaluation shows that you have advanced vessel disease, you won't have to resort to drugs at all. You will have controlled your cholesterol in a completely natural way.

Finally, Scenarios 1 and 2 could be reversed. The usual sequence would be first diet and exercise, then functional foods, and finally drugs. But there's nothing wrong with starting with a functional food—as both Scott and Adam did—and then moving back to diet and exercise.

Also, some people who simply can't get on track with a consistent diet-and-exercise program may actually start with drugs. Adam was on the verge of taking this route until he stumbled upon Benecol. But then those who actually begin to take medications may find that by utilizing one of the first two natural scenarios, they can begin to reduce their drug dosage—or even eliminate it.

We'll deal with drugs—and how to combine them with functional foods—in more detail in chapter 7. All you need to keep in mind now is that with the right use of nutriceuticals, you may not have to resort to prescription medications at all.

6

Scientific Support for Functional Foods

I'm quite confident and excited about recommending some of the new cholesterol-lowering functional foods to my patients—for one major reason: the scientific support for them is overwhelming.

The Classic Benecol Study

The classic study that confirmed the potency of Benecol—which contains a plant stanol ester as the operative ingredient, and has paved the way for other designed functional foods—was a 1995 report published in the prestigious *New England Journal of Medicine* (vol. 333, Nov. 16, 1995, pp. 1308–12).

Finnish investigators—led by Tatu A. Miettinen of the University of Helsinki—conducted a one-year study involving 153 men and women, randomly selected in the province of North Karelia, Finland. The participants, who ranged in age from 25 to 64, had mildly elevated cholesterol levels. (The study required that an individual's total cholesterol measurement be higher than 216.)

The subjects were divided into two groups, one of which consisted of 51 "controls" who consumed margarine *without* the sitostanol ester. The total cholesterol and "bad" LDL cholesterol values of those in this group can be found in the column in chart 4 labeled "Control Group—No stanol" (see page 99).

Another group of 102 participants ate margarine *with* the operative plant stanol ester. Of those assigned to this second group, one segment consumed 2.6 grams of the plant stanol ester product each day for the first six months. Then they ate 1.8 grams per day for the second six months. (This subgroup is included in the chart in the "1.8 gm/day" column.)

Another segment of this second group ate 2.6 grams of the plant extract per day for the *entire* 12-month period. (The results from this subgroup are reflected in the chart in the "2.6 gm/day" column.)

All of the groups were put on the control margarine (containing no plant stanol) for the first six weeks. After that the control group stayed with the control margarine, but the two plant stanol groups were given margarine containing their designated amounts of the plant stanol extract each day for the next 12 months.

During the study's one-year period, cholesterol levels in the control group remained about the same. But some dramatic changes occurred among the participants who were taking the margarine-plus-sitostanol.

Overall, these functional food groups experienced on average a 10.2 percent reduction in their total blood cholesterol, and a 14.1 percent decrease in the "bad" LDL cholesterol.

Will consuming more of the functional food result in a greater drop in cholesterol?

Common sense would say, "Of course!" But scientists know that common sense doesn't always apply in medical research. For example, there may be a dosage threshold, beyond which a particular substance doesn't work as well. But in this particular case, we find that common sense *would* be right—at least as far as the amounts tested were concerned.

In other words, when you break down the specific performance results for each of the plant extract groups, it becomes evident that *consuming more* of the functional food resulted in a *greater reduction* in cholesterol than eating the smaller amount. The chart shows how we reach this conclusion.

First, you identify blood values at the point when the participants began taking the plant extract margarine (after the initial six-week period of consuming the control margarine). Then you check the values at the end of the 12-month trial period.

This simple observation shows us that the group taking 1.8 grams per day experienced a decline in total cholesterol of only 7.8 percent. On the other hand, the group consuming 2.6 grams per day had a 10.2 percent decrease.

The differences in the percentage decreases for "bad" LDL cholesterol were even more marked. From the time they began the functional food to the end of the 12-month study, the 1.8-gram group saw a 9.8 percent decrease. In contrast, the 2.6-gram subjects enjoyed a much higher, 16.3 percent drop.

Chart 4 allows you to follow the sequence of these and other changes in total and "bad" LDL cholesterol among all groups during the 12-month study.

The All-Important Ratio Result

Perhaps the most striking finding of all in this study is that the extremely important ratio of total cholesterol to "good" HDL cholesterol improved dramatically for both of the functional food groups.

CHART 4

Total Cholesterol and "Bad" LDL Cholesterol

In Three Finnish Study Groups

Cholesterol test dates	Two Groups Taking Plant Stanol		Control Group
	1.8 gm/day	2.6 gm/day	No stanol
Total cholesterol			
6 weeks before start of study	236±4	235±4	237±5
Start of study	232±4	234±4	235±4
6 months	211±4	215±3	237±4
12 months (end of study)	214±4	210±4	210±4
14 months (2 mos. after end)	233±4	236±5	243±5
LDL cholesterol			
6 weeks before start of study	156±3	159±4	159±4
Start of study	153±4	160±4	159±4
6 months	137±3	141±4	160±4
12 months (end of study)	138±3	134±3	157±4
14 months (2 mos. after end)	160±4	153±5	164±4

(Source: *New England Journal of Medicine*, vol. 333, Nov. 16, 1995, p. 1310)

A major reason for this result is that the functional food lowered total cholesterol *without* affecting the participants' HDL levels. (The HDL findings, which I'll be referring to at various times, are not shown in chart 4, but are taken from the actual *New England Journal of Medicine* report.)

Specifically, here's how the ratios changed for each of the two functional food groups:

- Those taking the *lower* amounts of the plant stanol (1.8 gm/day) started with an average ratio of 4.07 and dropped to 3.69 by the end of the study.

- Those on the *higher* amounts of the plant stanol (2.6 gm/day) experienced a ratio decline from 4.42 to 3.96.

This latter ratio result is particularly noteworthy because, as you'll recall from chart 1 on page 30, a ratio of 4.42 would put a man without a history of cardiovascular disease in the "borderline" risk category, and a woman at the "high" risk level. But with the drop of 3.96, a man would be in the "acceptable" range, and a woman would make it to the "borderline" category.

Beating the Averages

Keep in mind that the changes in cholesterol values and ratios in this research report are expressed as *averages* for the study group. This means that some of the participants experienced lower percentage drops in their total and LDL cholesterol, while others enjoyed much higher decreases than the average.

Can you beat the averages?

To check how your body might respond to a designed functional food like Benecol—which was the margarine used in this study—you should have a cholesterol blood test done just prior to taking this nutriceutical. As indicated in Chapter 2, all the pertinent components and sub-components should be checked: total cholesterol, "bad" LDL cholesterol, "good" HDL cholesterol, and the ratio of total to HDL cholesterol.

The test should also report your triglyceride values. Even though these are typically not affected by a plant stanol ester, you may be one of those lucky few who do experience a drop—even a substantial drop—in triglycerides. A blood test can alert you to any peculiarities in your personal biochemistry.

Then have your blood cholesterol checked once again after about three weeks. (In fact, most benefits of Benecol appear for most people after only two to three weeks.) You may be pleasantly surprised to find that you're one of those people whose cholesterol responds much better than the average!

More Benefits

By now, you have a good idea of the important findings in this landmark Finnish study of Benecol. But I've been able to tease out other hidden benefits that my patients or I can use.

Take another look at chart 4, and you'll find these additional "nuggets," which should be useful to you as you formulate fresh strategies to bring your cholesterol under control the natural way.

Nugget 1: The Existence of a Compound Effect When a Low-Fat Diet Is Linked to a Functional Food

You'll note that total cholesterol dropped slightly in *all three groups* after they had taken the control margarine for the first six weeks.

This response apparently reflects the fact that the control margarine—even though it didn't contain the plant stanol—had lower amounts of saturated fat than spreads in the participants' regular diet. Butter, which is quite high in saturated fat, has traditionally been the spread of choice in Finland.

To put this another way, the low-fat part of the basic diet lowered the cholesterol starting point for the study participants. As a result, when they added the functional food, they got even more of a benefit because they had a kind of head start in maximizing their lipid control. Low-fat foods, eaten in conjunction with functional foods, will almost always produce a significant Compound Effect.

Nugget 2: A Short-Term Functional Food Carryover Effect

Another interesting point that emerges from this chart is that the total cholesterol and LDL cholesterol measurements of the participants consistently returned to pretreatment levels within two months after they stopped eating the margarine.

In fact, others who have used Benecol and similar products have found that their cholesterol reverts to baseline readings after just a few days.

The main message seems to be this: *To get the full effect, you must eat the nutriceutical regularly.* If you stop, the benefits disappear.

Nugget 3: A Three-Way Cholesterol-Lowering Effect from Functional Foods like Benecol

From studies such as the one described above, scientists have concluded that products like Benecol can reduce your total cholesterol and "bad" LDL cholesterol in three distinct ways:

First, as we've already seen, the plant stanol blocks absorption of dietary cholesterol through the small intestine walls by means of an internal biological mechanism. It also stops reabsorption of cholesterol that comes into the intestines through the bile produced by the liver.

Second, the Benecol products are designed to contain fewer calories than comparable spreads and salad dressings, so you are less likely to gain extra weight in body fat, which can hike your total and LDL cholesterol levels.

Third, the plant stanol margarine has a healthier composition of fat than regular margarine or butter. The nutriceutical spread is high in monounsaturated fats, which alone have been shown to lower cholesterol. The Benecol-type products also tend to be quite low in saturated fat, whereas margarine is higher, and butter is extremely high. This distinction is important because saturated fats—even when they contain no cholesterol—have been associated with an increase in cholesterol in the bloodstream.

Here's how the calories and saturated-fat numbers work out in the three different products—Benecol spread, regular margarine, and butter.

One 8-gram serving of the regular Benecol spread—which was the type employed in this study—has only 45 calories. Only 0.5 grams come from saturated fat. Furthermore, one serving of the "light" Benecol spread has just 30 calories, with no saturated-fat calories.

In contrast, an equivalent amount of regular margarine contains about 1.4 grams of saturated fat and has about 71 calories. The caloric content of a comparable serving of butter is about the same as that of margarine, but the amount of saturated fat is much higher—almost 5 grams.

Furthermore, the negative impact of the fats in a product like stick margarine may be even worse because of the presence of the substance known as *trans fats*.

A reminder on trans fats: There is a growing tendency in some scientific circles to warn against excessive consumption of so-called trans fats, which are produced during the hydrogenation process. You'll recall that hydrogenation involves the chemical transformation of fatty oils into saturated hard fats so that they can be used more easily in cooking and storage. I caution all my patients about these fats.

Filling in the Scientific Gaps

What are some of the other ways that Benecol and related products may help those with cholesterol concerns? Here are some findings from recent scientific investigations.

Extra Punch in Lowering Mildly Elevated Cholesterol. Benecol products may be able to reduce cholesterol levels in people with mildly elevated levels of cholesterol (hypercholesterolemia) even more than we have been led to believe.

That's the implication of a study conducted by Dr. Tu T. Nguyen of the Mayo Clinic (presented at a conference on cardiovascular disease prevention in Kensington Town Hall, London, Sept. 29–Oct. 2, 1998).

The 36 men and 43 women subjects began the study with an average total cholesterol of 232 and LDL of 153. Dr. Nguyen and his fellow researchers found that after 8 weeks, participants taking 3 grams per day of plant stanols through the American version of the Benecol spread had lowered their total cholesterol by an average of 22 percent and also their "bad" LDL cholesterol by 22 percent. Those taking only 2 grams per day had a 14 percent reduction in their total cholesterol and a 13 percent drop in their LDL.

Aiding Adults with Normal Cholesterol Levels. Even if you have achieved an "acceptable" classification of your cholesterol level, you can still derive benefits from a plant stanol margarine, according to a January 1997 report in the *Scandinavian Journal of Nutrition* (vol. 41, pp. 9–12).

Over a five-week period, the Finnish researchers in this investigation gave a plant stanol ester margarine to a group of adults, who began with average total cholesterol of 197. At the study's end, their average cholesterol had dropped to 166—and virtually the entire decline resulted from a decrease in "bad" LDL cholesterol.

You might ask, "Why lower cholesterol in a person with normal lipid levels?"

One reason is that a reading of 197 is *barely* "acceptable," according to the risk chart on page 30. Taking your measurements down toward the "low" category is even more desirable.

So a better question might be: "Why not lower your levels down to the 'low' risk range?" By the standards established by the risk chart, a "low" risk measurement would be below 180 mg/dl.

Also, many people with normal total cholesterol may be at borderline or high risk in other ways, perhaps because their "good" HDL levels are low—thus giving them a "high" risk ratio. If they can lower their total cholesterol, they may be able to bring their ratio down to an "acceptable" level, despite their low levels of HDL.

A Natural Treatment for Diabetics with High Cholesterol. Accelerated rates of atherosclerosis, with an increase in the risk for cardiovascular disease and heart attack, are common among diabetic patients—and functional foods may be an answer to their dilemma.

According to a 1994 Finnish study (*Diabetologia,* vol.

37, pp. 773–80), products containing plant stanol esters are effective in lowering cholesterol for patients with non–insulin dependent diabetes (NIDDM).

Don't Forget the Sterol Story. It's appropriate at this juncture for us to remember the description in chapter 4 of the research done at the Unilever Research Laboratorium in the Netherlands, and published in 1998 in the *European Journal of Clinical Nutrition*. The researchers in that study concluded that margarine, such as Take Control, containing sterol esters from soybean oil is as effective as margarine made with plant stanol esters (vol. 52, no. 5, May 1998, pp. 334–43).

These findings go hand in glove with the plant stanol research involving Benecol. For one thing, even though the processes for producing the extracts are different, the biochemical operations of the stanols and sterols are apparently similar. In other words, we can currently assume that the products operate through similar biological mechanisms to block the absorption of cholesterol into the bloodstream through the intestines.

Consequently, the stanol- and sterol-based functional foods are probably interchangeable for purposes of preparing a nutriceutical menu.

The uses of cholesterol-lowering functional foods are sure to continue to multiply as further research emerges. But a few questions still remain: What about the side effects? Is it possible that consuming these new products may have long-term negative health consequences?

Is It Really True There Are No Side Effects?

Fortunately, the rather extensive studies conducted so far have established that eating designed functional foods will produce no side effects. But a few qualifications should be kept in mind as you put together your own functional food strategy.

Qualification 1: Stick with the Recommended Doses of the Functional Foods

Scientists reported back in 1977 that taking very large doses of plant sterols—18 grams daily for three years—caused a few cases of constipation. But even in these megadoses, most of the study participants experienced no side effects.

And remember: The more recent studies—which have tested the Benecol products and similar nutriceuticals being produced for the general market—involve the consumption of only about 3 to 4.5 grams of plant stanol esters per day. (See *Canadian Journal of Physiology and Pharmacology,* vol. 75, 1997, pp. 217–27.)

I recommend that you stick to the relatively small doses recommended on the product labels. I find many times that patients become so enthusiastic about a new treatment or technique that they overdo it. You can run too much, diet too much—or eat too much of a functional food.

Of course, if your physician decides you should consume more, and you undergo regular medical monitoring, consuming larger amounts would be acceptable.

Qualification 2: Maintain a Healthy Intake of Foods Containing Beta-Carotene

Some people may experience mild reductions in blood levels of carotenoids after taking functional foods containing plant sterols or stanols, according to the 1998 *European Journal of Clinical Nutrition* study, conducted by J. S. Weststrate and G. W. Meijer (vol. 52, pp. 334–43).

Research has shown that carotenoids, such as beta-carotene, may be able to lower the risk of certain cancers through an antioxidant effect in the body. But I really don't regard the relatively modest reductions that may occur in blood carotenoids from these functional foods as anything to worry about.

In any case, whether you're taking a functional food or not, it's always wise to keep your daily intake of beta-carotene up to these levels:

You can obtain the one-day's minimum requirement that I have recommended for several years—about 25,000 IU, or "international units"—by eating 1½ medium-size carrots or a medium-size sweet potato. Those who can't get at least 25,000 IU per day of beta-carotene through foods should make up the difference with a supplement.

To sum up, I am quite comfortable recommending such functional foods to adults with elevated or unbalanced cholesterol because the research confirming the benefits is highly convincing—and the possibility of side effects is remote. Please note that McNeil Consumer Healthcare—producer of Benecol—cautions that pregnant women should consult with their physician before making any dietary change, and I agree this is wise advice.

But what about possible side effects for the traditional functional foods—especially grains, which contain soluble fiber? Again, the chance of a negative reaction is remote, but there are a number of facts that all patients should know—especially those with allergies.

What About Side Effects with the Traditional Foods?

As with the designed products, the traditional functional foods, such as those made from psyllium and oat products, are highly unlikely to cause you any health problems. But because a few people do have certain negative reactions—most of them allergic—I want to provide you with a summary of possible symptoms and dangers.

Psyllium products, including cereals and laxatives, may, in rare instances, trigger a severe allergic reaction known as *anaphylaxis,* which can be fatal unless immediate medical attention is given. Here are some illustrations:

- A 39-year-old nurse with a history of nasal and eye symptoms after exposure to psyllium, developed anaphylaxis after taking an over-the-counter psyllium bulk laxative. Her symptoms: flushing; excessively fast heartbeat (tachycardia); welts on the skin (urticaria); swelling of the larynx (laryngeal edema); swelling of the skin and mucous membranes (angioedema); and lightheadedness. (See *Allergy Proceedings,* vol. 11, Sept.–Oct. 1990, pp. 241–42.)

- A 38-year-old woman developed anaphylaxis 25 minutes after having a psyllium-containing breakfast cereal. She experienced hypotension (low blood pressure), a feeling of constriction in the throat, hoarseness, dyspnea (shortness of breath), wheezing, generalized pruritus (itching), urticaria (skin blotches and welts), and vomiting.

    But she recovered completely after being treated with epinephrine, normal saline, diphenhydramine, and methylprednisolone. (See *American Journal of Emergency Medicine,* vol. 9, Sept. 1991, pp. 449–51.)

- Cereals containing oats, wheat, rye, and barley may trigger allergic reactions in some people. A wise preventive measure for those with any allergy symptoms related to these products is to consult an allergy specialist, who may order a variety of tests, including the prick test, the RAST, and the histamine-release test. (See *Allergy,* vol. 49, Dec. 1994, pp. 871–76.)

• Exercise after consumption of a cereal may produce allergic reactions or even anaphylaxis in some people. (See *Clinical Experiments in Allergy,* vol. 27, Feb. 1997, pp. 162–66.) But this is a rare response.

Although I want you to be aware of these possible negative reactions that may occur in a few people after they eat cereals—including those containing soluble fiber—I certainly don't want to scare you away from these important functional foods. So keep in mind two important points:

• If you have a history of allergic reactions— especially to cereals—you should consult your physician and perhaps undergo additional tests before you increase your intake of these foods.

• If you or a family member should develop any of the symptoms listed above—especially those suggesting anaphylaxis—you should immediately head for the emergency room. This sort of allergic reaction, which may also occur in some people after a bee sting or eating some other food, can be deadly. But if you get to the hospital or a clinic quickly and get the proper treatment, you'll recover completely.

To sum up, the medical establishment has confirmed that Benecol and related products work quite well on those with:

• elevated total cholesterol;

• elevated "bad" LDL cholesterol;

- normal total cholesterol—especially when this measurement is accompanied by low "good" HDL levels (a condition that will result in a higher total-to-HDL ratio, which can significantly raise cardio-vascular risk);

- non–insulin dependent diabetes mellitus plus high cholesterol; and

- patients taking cholesterol-lowering drugs, who want to reduce the doses of their medications—or in some cases, completely eliminate the need for the drugs.

To expand further on this final point, let's turn now to a consideration of the cholesterol-lowering medications that are currently available—and how they can be combined with functional foods in a wise strategy for controlling cholesterol.

7

The Drug Connection: Combining Medications with Functional Foods

A revolution that promises to shake the foundations of modern medical practice is now emerging for those of us who treat high cholesterol with prescription drugs.

We finally are acquiring the knowledge and developing the tools we need to help people who simply can't handle normal doses of cholesterol-lowering drugs. As a possible forerunner of cholesterol treatment in the future, let's consider the situation of Kevin, who relied on functional foods to achieve minimal doses of his statin medications.

Kevin's Satisfying Statin Story

Kevin's blood fats certainly didn't look promising for low-dose drug therapy when he started out. His total cholesterol measured 340, and his "good" HDL cholesterol was low at 41—a combination that gave him an undesirable, high-risk ratio of 8.29.

But then he embarked seriously on a low-fat diet. (See the description of Scenario 1 on page 91.) As a result, he succeeded in bringing his total cholesterol down to 290. Also, by increasing his weekly endurance exercise, he managed to raise his HDL level to 42—and consequently lower his ratio to 6.9.

As yet Kevin had no symptoms of cardiovascular disease, such as angina pains or an abnormal stress test. But the results of an Ultrafast CT scan revealed that he had significant calcification of his arteries—or a buildup of plaque that is a sign of vessel disease.

He knew he had to do a better job of lowering his total cholesterol and balancing his overall blood-lipid profile, or he would probably end up taking relatively high drug doses. So he moved into the next stage of his battle— functional foods (Scenario 2).

After using a Benecol plant stanol ester spread for two to three weeks, Kevin had his cholesterol tested again and found these changes:

- Total cholesterol had declined to 258.

- HDL levels remained the same at 42.

- Ratio of total cholesterol to HDL cholesterol had dropped to 6.15.

These changes certainly put him in a better position. But given the tendency of his arteries to become blocked by the buildup of oxidized LDL cholesterol, his physician recommended medications.

At this point, Kevin had a number of options—which we'll discuss in some detail shortly. But his physician chose one of the statin drugs, simvastatin (brand name: Zocor), which helped him reach a final resolution to his cholesterol problem.

He began to take Zocor in daily doses that were much smaller than he would have required if he had failed to take the first two steps in the strategy. Within a few weeks, his total cholesterol had declined once again, this time to 177. Also, his "good" HDL cholesterol went up a notch to 43.

Now the ratio of Kevin's total cholesterol to HDL cholesterol was down to an "acceptable" level of 4.12.

Because of the impact of the dietary changes and the functional food on his cholesterol, Kevin was able to operate on extremely low doses of his statin drug—so low, in fact, that there was virtually no chance of any side effects.

Kevin's experience bodes well for future treatment, as physicians begin to combine functional foods with statins—and discover that they can lower drug doses or eliminate them completely. I certainly applaud the advent of this new mode of treatment.

What Was Happening in Kevin's Body?

Researchers have discovered that with a patient like Kevin, combining medications with certain functional foods—especially those like Benecol with plant stanol esters—can produce a kind of *synergistic effect.* In other words, the functional food not only adds an outside lipid-lowering factor on top of the normal operation of the drug, but it may also actually increase the inherent power of the drug to lower cholesterol.

Here are a few representative findings, which undoubtedly will be replicated in the months and years ahead:

• A synergistic effect in lowering cholesterol occurred in women with previous heart attacks when simvastatin (Zocor) was combined with a sitostanol ester margarine (Benecol), according to rescarchers Helena Gylling and her colleagues from the University of Helsinki. (See *Circulation*, vol. 96, Dec. 16, 1997, pp. 4226–31.)

The precise explanation of how this synergism—or mutually empowering interaction between drugs and plant stanols—works involves understanding some rather complex biochemical processes and concepts. But here's my best attempt to simplify the findings:

The researchers determined that patients who are on a statin drug (which inhibits synthesis of cholesterol in the body) may be at a disadvantage if they also absorb too much cholesterol through the intestinal wall. The reason: The drug may be overwhelmed by excessive amounts of cholesterol that enter the bloodstream through the intestines.

But taking a functional food containing a plant stanol ester *in addition to* the statin drug introduces a mechanism that inhibits absorption of the cholesterol in the bile at the intestinal level. The functional food, through its blocking action in the intestines, reduces the cholesterol that reenters the bloodstream. This limits the cholesterol to manageable levels for the drug and enables the drug to bring the remaining blood cholesterol down to a normal range.

In effect, then, the use of the drug and the functional food together produced a two-plus-two effect that equaled more than four—or accomplished more than what either mode of treatment could have achieved independently.

• A similar synergistic effect—with an exponential increase in cholesterol-lowering power—occurred when another statin drug, pravastatin (Pravachol), was combined with a sitostanol ester margarine (Benecol). (See *Journal of Lipid Research,* vol. 37, 1996, pp. 1776–85.)

In this study, conducted with eight diabetic men with high cholesterol, participants took the pravastatin with the functional food margarine, which contained 3 grams per day of sitostanol ester.

The result was that their "bad" LDL cholesterol was lowered on average by 44 percent during the seven-week study. Also, the researchers noted that the combination treatment was safe and should enable many patients to go on lower doses of the drug.

• In another 1994 report from the University of Helsinki, researcher H. Vanhanen determined that total cholesterol values among certain patients were not being reduced sufficiently by pravastatin (Pravachol) alone. As a result, he looked to other ways to control the blood lipid. (See *European Journal of Clinical Nutrition,* vol. 47, 1994, pp. 169–176.)

Noting that pravastatin works by inhibiting the synthesis of cholesterol in the liver, Vanhanen decided to add a treatment that would work through another biological mechanism—namely, interference with the absorption of cholesterol into the bloodstream through the intestines. The two methods chosen for testing were the powerful prescription antibiotic neomycin, and a product containing a sitostanol ester (developed by Raisio, the Finnish company that produces Benecol).

The conclusion: The neomycin-pravastatin combination very effectively inhibited both cholesterol synthesis and absorption of cholesterol into the bloodstream. The sitostanol ester also worked, but in this case not as well as the antibiotic.

But what happens when you put the antibiotic neomycin and a plant-stanol functional food together? Check the next item.

● A 1995 study published in *Atherosclerosis* revealed that combining neomycin with a sitostanol ester margarine (Benecol) resulted in a 37 percent reduction in the blood concentrations of both total and "bad" LDL cholesterol. According to the researchers, this drop reflected almost total inhibition of cholesterol absorption through the intestine. (See *Atherosclerosis,* vol. 117, 1995, pp. 305–308.)

From these and other studies, it has become increasingly obvious that, whenever possible, an effective cholesterol-lowering functional food should be taken with medications. But whatever individual or combination technique you use, your goal must be lowering your elevated cholesterol as quickly as you can—because your life depends on it.

Understanding the Combination Strategy

Getting your elevated cholesterol down to normal levels may require some kind of prescription medication—even if the presence of functional foods means that the drug can be taken in lower doses than in the past. So what are the basic drugs—and how can they be used most effectively with functional foods to help you establish control over your cholesterol? Let's launch this discussion with a summary of how functional foods and lifestyle changes can be combined most effectively with a strategy that combines nutriceuticals and other natural measures with drug therapy. Then we'll take a look at specific drugs.

If you have a cholesterol problem, your primary objective should be to find a way to control your blood fats *without* drugs—as quickly as possible. Because functional foods are such great incentives for launching a successful, full-scale cholesterol-lowering program, I've included them in the first two steps. Then the lifestyle approaches follow, and finally the medications.

Each step includes percentage estimates for cholesterol reduction. It's *extremely important,* by the way, that you go through *all* of these steps. If you omit any of them, you'll lose the chance for the indicated percentage benefit—and increase the likelihood that your drug dose will increase. And when you move on to another step, you should continue following the previous step or steps. Only by adding new steps to previous ones can you enjoy the full compound effect.

....

The Nutriceutical-Drug Combination Strategy

Step 1: Reduce your total cholesterol by *10 percent* or more and your "bad" LDL cholesterol by *14 percent* or more by eating recommended daily servings of a designed functional food, such as Benecol or Take Control.

Step 2: Reduce your total cholesterol by *5 percent* with a traditional functional food, such as a cereal with high quantities of psyllium.

Step 3: Reduce your total cholesterol by *15 percent* or more with a low-fat, low-cholesterol diet.

The total fat calories in your diet should constitute no more than 25 percent of total daily calories, and saturated fat calories should be no more than 8 percent of total calories. Your diet should also include no more than 200 mg per day of cholesterol.

Step 4: Raise your "good" HDL cholesterol by *10 percent* or more through regular endurance exercise.

If you aren't currently exercising, or if you are only a sporadic exerciser, here's a suggestion for a simple HDL-raising aerobics program: For 1 month, walk as fast as you can for 20 continuous minutes, 3 days per week. After 1 month, gradually increase your walking time to 30 minutes, and your number of weekly sessions to 4.

Step 5: Lower your total cholesterol by *5 percent* for every 5 to 10 pounds you lose in excess body weight.

Step 6 (if necessary): Lower your total cholesterol by *25 percent* or more, and your "bad" LDL cholesterol by *30 percent* or more with statin drugs.

Alternative Step 6 (if necessary): Use a combination of a statin drug plus a bile acid sequestrant to increase the reduction of your "bad" LDL cholesterol by 45 percent or more.

Step 7 (if necessary): Use a special triglyceride-lowering drug, such as atorvastatin (Lipitor), to lower *triglycerides by 30 percent* or more.

....

Now here's a quick illustration of how these steps and their percentages might work in a woman with rather "bad numbers" on a cholesterol report.

Assume that this patient—"Rachel"—is in her early forties and hasn't yet gone through menopause. Her total cholesterol is 290; her "bad" LDL cholesterol, 220; her "good" HDL, 39; and her total-to-HDL ratio, 7.44. As you can see, she is at a "high" risk level in all categories, as indicated in chart 1 on page 30.

If Rachel can't change those numbers, I would recommend that she go on a cholesterol-lowering drug—and so would most other doctors I know. I might choose simvastatin (Zocor), which is usually prescribed in doses ranging from 10 to 80 mg daily. But in her case, the dose would most likely have to be considerably higher than the minimum to bring her total and LDL cholesterol down into the acceptable ranges.

But if Rachel moves through each step in the nutriceutical-drug strategy, her drug situation could be entirely different. Here's what might happen, just to her total and HDL cholesterol:

Step 1: With a designed functional food like Benecol, her total cholesterol could drop by 10 percent to 261.

Step 2: With a traditional functional food, such as Kellogg's Bran Buds, her total cholesterol could drop by another 5 percent to 248.

Step 3: With a low-fat, low-cholesterol diet, her total cholesterol could decrease by another 15 percent to 211.

Step 4: With aerobic exercise, her "good" HDL cholesterol should rise by 10 percent to 43.

Step 5: With a 10-pound weight loss, her total cholesterol probably would decline by 5 percent to 200.

Now, we've reached the steps that involve drugs—but let's evaluate Rachel's status. Her total cholesterol is 200, and her "good" HDL cholesterol is 43—results that give her a ratio of 4.66.

Clearly, Rachel has made great progress—but still, her lipids need work. She is right on the line between the "borderline" and "acceptable" categories for total cholesterol; in the "borderline" range for HDL cholesterol; and "high" for her ratio.

Should she go on drugs with these measurements?

The question is harder to answer than it would be if she had done nothing to control her cholesterol naturally. Most likely, if she has no other cardiovascular risk factors, I would say forget the drugs at this point and urge her to keep working on lowering her cholesterol through more stringent diet and weight loss. Also, she should try to raise her HDL still higher through exercise.

On the other hand, if Rachel has two or more additional cardiovascular risk factors, such as high blood pressure, I might recommend the smallest dose of simvastatin (Zocor)—perhaps even less than the usual 10-mg minimum (such as a 5-mg dose).

Clearly, then, with Rachel the nutriceutical-drug combination strategy makes a great deal of sense. In fact, she might well be able to eliminate the drugs altogether.

For those who have to go on drugs, even if they are low doses, I've included a brief overview below of the major cholesterol-controlling drugs that are being prescribed by many doctors. You can use this as a kind of "Patient's Desk Reference" if you find you have to include drugs in your combination strategy.

A Quick Guide to the Four Basic Cholesterol Drugs—And Further Tips on Combining Them with Functional Foods

Four basic types of cholesterol-lowering drugs are commonly used by doctors today—and are combined with the natural forms of lipid therapy. These include (1) statins, (2) bile acid sequestrants, (3) fibric acid derivatives, and (4) nicotinic acid (or niacin).

While a doctor's prescription is required for the first three, the fourth—niacin—is available over the counter. But *all four categories* should be treated as drugs and should be taken only under the supervision of a qualified physician.

Here are some details about how each type of drug operates in your body, plus possible side effects. Even as I list these possible side effects, however, I don't want to scare you away from a cholesterol-lowering medication you may need. Don't forget the key point about these medications: There is plenty of evidence that reducing your total cholesterol level to a low-risk range—and otherwise balancing your cholesterol subcomponents, such as LDL and HDL—will greatly reduce your risk of cardiovascular disease and premature death.

Just stay in close touch with your doctor when you go on one of these drugs, and undergo regular basic health exams, such as those blood tests that evaluate your various liver functions. In this way, you'll be able to stop the drug in plenty of time if serious side effects show up.

If anything, the possibility of experiencing side effects from these medications should motivate you to pay even closer attention to the first two scenarios. (See pages 91–92.) You'll recall that they focus on natural programs such as a low-fat diet, endurance exercise, and functional foods—such as the plant stanol and sterol products, and soluble fiber. The more success you experience with these powerful nonpharmacological approaches to controlling your cholesterol, the more likely it is that you'll be able to take relatively low drug doses—or eliminate the need for medications altogether.

The Statins

Statins—also known by the technical name *HMG-CoA reductase inhibitors*—encompass a wide range of relatively new medications that prevent the synthesis of "bad" LDL cholesterol in the liver. They also improve the body's power to remove LDL molecules from the blood by encouraging the development and operation of *LDL receptors*. These receptors, which are situated in the liver and on the vessel walls, in effect "catch" the loose LDL in the blood and remove it from circulation.

Statins are more effective than other types of drugs currently on the market in lowering levels of total and LDL cholesterol in the blood. Typically, they lower LDL by at least 25 to 30 percent, and they may reduce its levels by as much as 40 to 60 percent.

So if you can get your LDL cholesterol only down to 190 through a low-fat diet and functional foods, adding a statin drug to your program could take you down at least to the 140 range. In fact, it's likely that you'll make it to about 115, or even to a level below 100.

But remember: To get down to these low levels, you should first do all you can to decrease your total and bad cholesterol through lifestyle adjustments and functional foods. Only then should you turn to a statin drug—which at that point you will probably be able to take in smaller doses.

The statins may also raise "good" HDL levels by around 10 percent, and they can lower triglycerides—the other important and potentially destructive blood fat—by about 20 percent.

Some of the popular statins include:

- simvastatin (Zocor);

- lovastatin (Mevacor);

- pravastatin (Pravachol); and

- atorvastatin (Lipitor).

The typical daily dose of these drugs is 10 to 80 mg daily; the dose is determined by the patient's cholesterol level, cardiovascular risk, and response to the medication. The dose is usually taken in the evening. There's a good reason for this timing: Most cholesterol production in the body takes place between midnight and 3:00 A.M. As a result, the statins, which are designed to disrupt the LDL synthesis process, should be in the body before the early "cholesterol-manufacturing" mechanism in the liver gets into full operation.

Conversely, some of the effectiveness of these drugs (except Lipitor) will be lost if they are taken in the morning. Lipitor can be taken at any time during the day. (See *The Medical Letter: On Drugs and Therapeutics,* vol. 35, no. 891, March 5, 1993, pp. 19–22.)

My own current practice with these drugs can be summed up this way:

- If a patient has elevated total cholesterol that can't be reduced to an acceptable level by lifestyle strategies and nutriceuticals, I prescribe 10 mg of simvastatin (Zocor), to be taken at night.

- If the patient has a combination of high triglycerides (over 200), low "good" HDL cholesterol (below about 35), and elevated total cholesterol (above the 240 level), I may prescribe atorvastatin (Lipitor).

Most of my patients have found that in these low doses, they suffer few, if any, side effects. But if you happen to be one of those unlucky people who happens to run into a problem, you should know the danger signals and what to do about them.

Side Effects The statin drugs usually cause fewer side effects than other cholesterol-lowering drugs, and that's one of the main reasons for their recent rise in popularity.

Possible adverse reactions from the statins include gastrointestinal disturbances (such as an upset stomach or unpleasant bowel movement alterations); skin rashes;

muscle aches; and headaches. Also, a few people suffer from interrupted sleep.

Rarely, in 1 to 2 percent of patients, there may be liver damage. For this reason, it's extremely important for anyone taking these drugs to have regular blood tests that measure liver function.

Also, in a few cases, patients have reported a lupuslike condition—including scaly changes in the skin and, in the worst situations, deterioration of internal organs.

There have also been infrequent reports of *myopathy,* or muscle disease accompanied by pains and other feelings of discomfort. Myopathy and other adverse reactions may also occur if you're taking a statin with other drugs, including cyclosporine (Sandimmune), gemfibrozil (Lopid), niacin, or erythromycin (an antibiotic).

Just stay in close touch with your doctor when you go on one of these drugs, and undergo regular basic health exams, such as those blood tests that evaluate your various liver functions. In this way, you'll be able to stop the drug in plenty of time if serious side effects show up.

Bile Acid Sequestrants

Another commonly used medication—which employs a completely different biological mechanism than the statins to lower your blood lipids—is the bile acid sequestrant.

Bile acid sequestrant drugs—which include cholestyramine (Questran and Questran Light) and colestipol (Colestid)—work by "binding" bile acids that return from the liver to the intestinal tract.

Since there are large amounts of cholesterol in the bile, this action of binding or tying up the bile prevents the bile cholesterol from circulating again through the walls of the small intestine and returning to the bloodstream. Instead, the cholesterol that is captured by the sequestrant is washed out of the body through the bowel movement.

Various studies have demonstrated that these drugs are so effective that they can lower "bad" LDL cholesterol by 15 to 30 percent. In the process, they lower total cholesterol and may also raise "good" HDL cholesterol by as much as 10 percent. Unfortunately, however, the sequestrants may also raise triglyceride levels in some patients.

The typical daily dosage for cholestyramine is 4 to 16 grams per day, with a maximum recommended daily dose of 24 grams. For colestipol, the usual dosage is 5 to 20 grams per day, with a maximum of 30 grams a day.

Although these drugs pose less danger to the liver than the statins, they must be monitored regularly because of their potential for raising triglycerides. Also, they can interfere with the absorption of other drugs. To guard against this problem, it's best to take the bile acid sequestrant one hour before, or four to six hours after, you take any other drug.

Note: Remember that the soluble fiber in traditional functional foods, such as oat and psyllium products, also lowers cholesterol by binding the bile. If you try both approaches at the same time, it's uncertain what the total effect might be because we lack studies on this point.

On one hand, because the soluble-fiber mechanism is so close to that of bile acid sequestrants, it may be that one or the other would have a lessened effect. On the other hand, by working together they might produce an enhanced synergistic effect. In any event, there's no risk associated with taking both together.

What I suggest for my patients in a situation like this is to conduct an experiment under your doctor's supervision. Check the impact of the two techniques on your own body by scheduling a cholesterol blood test while you're on the drug but immediately before you begin to take the soluble fiber. Then take another test about three weeks later, and see if your total or LDL cholesterol goes down or stays the same.

If your cholesterol goes down, you are most likely benefiting from a synergistic response—and should continue with both programs. If there is no change, the soluble fiber is probably being over-ridden by the drug, or vice versa. So there's evidently no need to rely on a soluble-fiber approach in this situation to lower your cholesterol.

Finally, keep in mind that here we're talking *only* about bile acid sequestrants and functional foods with soluble fiber. Other drugs, as well as designed functional foods such as Benecol, work by other biological mechanisms.

Side Effects Possible negative side effects of the sequestrants include constipation, rectal bleeding, stomach upsets, gas, and other gastrointestinal problems. After the body gets used to the drug, however, these effects tend to recede. Also, you can minimize the adverse reactions by taking the drugs just before mealtime.

To counter constipation, include extra amounts of insoluble fiber (such as wheat bran) in your diet. Extra soluble fiber can help as well. (As you can see, there may be reasons other than lowering cholesterol to up your intake of psyllium and oats!)

Fibrates

A class of drugs known as fibrates and fibric acid derivatives have been successful in lowering triglycerides, raising "good" HDL cholesterol, lowering total cholesterol, and sometimes reducing "bad" LDL.

One of these drugs, gemfibrozil (Lopid), which has been used by practicing physicians for many years, can lower triglycerides by 30 to 60 percent and can raise HDL cholesterol by 10 to 20 percent. The mechanism involves interfering with the synthesis of the dangerous lipid subfraction Apolipoprotein B (Apo B).

The normal dose of gemfibrozil is 600 mg twice a day, which should be taken 30 minutes before breakfast and 30 minutes before the evening meal. The maximum recommended dose is 1,500 mg daily.

Side Effects Possible adverse effects of many members of the fibrate family include stomach and upper gastrointestinal problems such as gas or nausea. Also, some patients experience myopathy—the weakening of the muscles, which may include muscle pains. In addition, there may be negative interactions with other drugs, including anticoagulants such as warfarin, and also the statins.

A note on probucol: At one time, probucol (Lorelco) also seemed to be a promising fibric acid derivative. It was effective in lowering total serum cholesterol and "bad" LDL cholesterol, but it had no effect on reducing triglycerides.

What made this drug lose favor with most clinicians was that it could lower "good" HDL cholesterol significantly and increase the all-important ratio of total cholesterol to HDL cholesterol. For that reason, probucol is not commonly used at this time.

A New Fibrate Family Member. Perhaps the newest member of this fibrate family is TriCor, which consists of fenofibrate capsules. This drug is used to treat adult patients with very high blood triglyceride levels who are at risk for pancreatitis (inflammation of the pancreas) and are not responding well to dietary efforts to control triglycerides. Typically, these patients have blood triglyceride levels in excess of 2,000 mg/dl. (Remember, the goal for those without heart or vessel disease is to get triglycerides below 151 and preferably below 125.)

Clinical trials have shown that this drug can lower total triglycerides by 50 percent and can raise HDL cholesterol by 35 percent. Total cholesterol may also decrease, but LDL cholesterol may go up. (See *Medical Letter: On Drugs and Therapeutics,* vol. 40, July 3, 1998, pp. 68–69.)

One study actually showed that a particular statin drug, atorvastatin (Lipitor), was less effective than fenofibrate in lowering triglyceride levels and raising HDL cholesterol. But the statin did a better job of lowering "bad" LDL cholesterol.

Current scientific thinking suggests that TriCor works by inhibiting the body's biological synthesis of triglycerides. The initial dose is usually 67 milligrams per day, with a maximum dose of three 67-mg capsules taken once per day with a meal.

Are There Drawbacks for TriCor? TriCor is not recommended for patients with liver, kidney, or gallbladder disease.

The most frequently reported adverse effects include infection, various pains, skin rashes, and flulike symptoms. Other possible negative reactions include an intensification of the effects of anticoagulant drugs, such as Coumadin. Some patients may experience myopathy (muscle disease with pain) and related problems.

Niacin

The over-the-counter drug nicotinic acid, or niacin (vitamin B_3), has long been known as an effective treatment to lower total and "bad" LDL cholesterol without lowering the "good" HDL cholesterol. In fact, with some people, niacin actually causes the HDL to rise.

But even though it is sold without a prescription, *niacin should always be regarded as a medication and should be taken only under the supervision of a physician.* This medication can be dangerous, in part because it's so seductive. Niacin is much cheaper than any of the other drugs, and it's readily available—as accessible as your supermarket or pharmacy shelf.

The biological mechanism by which niacin operates isn't entirely clear, but many experts feel that it interferes with the production of a particular kind of cholesterol—very low-density lipoprotein, or VLDL. Since the body's chemical processes convert VLDL into LDL, reducing the amount of VLDL will also reduce levels of "bad" LDL cholesterol.

Make no mistake about the pharmacological power of niacin. Studies have shown that it can lower LDL by 15 to 30 percent, raise HDL by 10 to 40 percent, and also lower triglycerides by 20 to 50 percent. This very potency is also a weakness from a medical point of view—primarily because of the dangers posed by such a readily available drug, which may not be monitored closely enough by a qualified physician.

But when properly supervised, patients may enjoy success. One 44-year-old woman who took 1 to 1.5 grams (1,000 to 1,500 mg) daily for a few months experienced a decrease in total cholesterol from 215 to 185, a drop of about 14 percent. Most of this resulted from a decrease of her "bad" LDL cholesterol. There was also a small beneficial effect on her "good" HDL cholesterol. Before the niacin treatment, her HDL cholesterol reading was naturally or genetically low, at 38. (It should have been above 69.) After the treatment, it rose to 43.

In this case, the niacin, by lowering the total cholesterol

while at the same time slightly elevating the HDL, improved the ratio of total to HDL cholesterol considerably. Before the medications, the patient had a ratio of 5.66—a figure that placed her in a very high-risk category for cardiovascular disease. But after taking the niacin, her ratio dropped to 4.30—still rather high for a woman her age, but nevertheless in a lower-risk category.

In general, niacin is taken in doses of 1.5 to 3 grams per day, though some patients have reported success with lower doses of about 1 gram per day. The higher the dose, the greater the risk of liver problems. But no more than 3 grams (3,000 mg) per day should be taken under any circumstances.

Side Effects Niacin is a drug—and should be taken only under the supervision of a physician. The reason for this warning is that some people have suffered liver damage after taking it. So anyone on niacin should undergo regular blood tests that check the liver function. Time-release niacin has been associated with more problems than regular niacin, and so I typically recommend the regular type for my patients.

Another problem with niacin is that it may cause histamine to be released in the body—a result that may cause problems for asthma patients.

One recent study has shown that higher dosages may actually cause a "backfire effect" by raising triglyceride levels. Also, higher levels greatly increase the risk of liver problems and other complications, such as increasing the homocysteine level. (Homocysteine, a by-product of the breakdown of an amino acid in the blood, can be measured in special blood tests and may be as good a predictor of cardiovascular risk as cholesterol.)

Even at lower doses, this powerful vitamin can cause uncomfortable side effects, including flushing, an upset stomach, and other gastrointestinal problems. Flushing, which usually goes away after a few weeks of use, can be minimized or prevented by taking an aspirin with the niacin tablet. Taking niacin with meals instead of on an empty stomach can usually eliminate GI symptoms.

What is my position, as a practicing physician, on niacin?

In the past, I've recommended the use of niacin by some patients. But in more recent years I've been leaning more toward prescribing statins instead because they have fewer side effects and risks. One drawback to the statins, of course, is that they cost considerably more than niacin. Recent estimates peg the minimum cost of statins at about $1,200 per year or more, and the outlay can go much higher if higher doses are required. In contrast, niacin typically costs less than $100 per year.

Fine-tuning the Medication Strategy

With this guide to the main cholesterol-managing drugs in hand, you and your physician may now be in a position to "get fancy" by enhancing the effect of two cholesterol medications by combining them in your treatment program.

In our discussion of the three scenarios on pages 91–95, you've seen how various cholesterol-lowering techniques can produce an exponential Compound Effect in your bloodstream and intestines. Functional foods, a low-fat diet, weight reduction, and exercise pile upon one another, lowering your cholesterol levels by a growing percentage through a variety of biological mechanisms.

But there are also ways that you can take advantage of this Compound Effect if your physician determines you must also go on drugs. For example, you might combine two drugs that operate through different biological mechanisms—with the result that you achieve a more powerful effect than you could get using just one drug.

You may also find that this double-drug approach, plus your natural program, actually helps you lower your total drug dose below the total dose for one drug alone.

That's what happened in a study published in 1995 in the *American Journal of Cardiology* (vol. 75, pp. 34–39). The report revealed that low-dose combination therapy with colestipol and a statin lowered cholesterol effectively—and at a reduced total cost for treatment.

In this investigation, the researchers found that patients who received 10 grams of the bile acid sequestrant colestipol (Colestid) plus 20 grams of lovastatin (Mevacor) experienced a 48 percent decrease in their "bad" LDL. Their average LDL levels dropped from 189 to 97.

This combination drug regimen was tolerated well by the participants, with the only significant side effects being constipation and some headaches. I don't hesitate to use such a strategy if a patient responds well to it.

Why You Haven't Failed If You Must Use a Drug

Many of my patients become discouraged when they find they have to take a cholesterol-controlling medication. They may try functional foods, a low-fat diet, and exercise, but they just can't seem to reduce their risk sufficiently.

In such cases, I emphasize that I certainly don't regard them as failures just because they haven't been able to eliminate drugs altogether.

My real test for success focuses on their answer to this

question: "Have I taken every natural step I possibly can to reduce my drug dose?"

If your answer is yes, that's all you can do. And you are a resounding success if you've lowered your original drug dose only slightly!

In addition to exploring with your physician the possibility of combining cholesterol medications, you should also keep in mind several additional advantages of some of the drugs that you may have to take.

Longer Life. A 5.4-year Scandinavian study of patients using simvastatin (Zocor) showed that the simvastatin patients enjoyed significantly improved survival rates over patients who didn't take a medication. (See *Lancet*, vol. 344, Nov. 19, 1994, pp. 1383–89.)

During the study, the participants on simvastatin enjoyed average drops in their total cholesterol of 25 percent and in their "bad" LDL cholesterol of 35 percent. Their "good" HDL cholesterol rose 8 percent on average.

The results for mortality and disease were even more dramatic. Zocor reduced total mortality (deaths) by 30 percent and coronary morality by 42 percent. Also, the drug lowered the need for coronary surgery by 37 percent and cut the incidence of coronary events, including nonfatal events, by 34 percent.

Reduced Stroke Risk. In 1997, researchers from the Harvard Medical School and several Boston hospitals analyzed various trials using statin drugs from 1985 to 1995 to see if the medications reduced the risks of stroke and total mortality. (See *JAMA*, vol. 278, no. 4, July 23–30, 1997, pp. 313–21.)

They concluded that the 16 trials they examined, which included about 29,000 subjects, confirmed that the average reduction in total cholesterol was 22 percent, and the average drop in "bad" LDL was 30 percent. Even more important, those on the statins experienced significant reductions of 29 percent in their risk of stroke, and 22 percent in risk of total mortality.

Lower Risk from Triglycerides. Recent reviews for atorvastatin (Lipitor) have focused on its ability to lower cardiovascular risk by lowering levels of triglycerides, the blood lipid that is a cousin to cholesterol.

A 1996 report in the *Journal of the American Medical Association* (vol. 275, Jan. 10, 1996, pp. 128–33) concluded that this drug was able to lower blood-triglyceride levels progressively as doses were increased. Specifically, triglycerides dropped over a 4-week treatment period by amounts that ranged on average from 26.5 to 46 percent, depending on the size of the dose. Furthermore, the patients tolerated the atorvastatin well, with few side effects.

Fewer Symptoms of Heart Disease. A report issued in 1998 suggested that Lipitor may not only lower cholesterol but may also reduce symptoms of heart disease and eliminate or delay the need for balloon angioplasty, which is an invasive procedure designed to open up clogged arteries. (See *Wall Street Journal,* Nov. 12, 1998, p. B6.)

In this study, announced at the 1998 American Heart Association meeting by the Warner-Lambert Company, the researchers found that 13 percent of patients treated with Lipitor suffered heart problems during the study period, as compared with 21 percent of patients who underwent angioplasty.

As for the impact on blood lipids, those taking Lipitor enjoyed an average decrease in "bad" LDL cholesterol from a starting level of 140 to an end point of 77—or well down into the lowest-risk range.

Experts commenting on this study said that among other things, the results show that doctors should do a better job of getting heart patients' LDL cholesterol below 100.

In summing up the impact of these and other advances, authors of a 1998 review of the state of the research into statins predicted that for every 10 percent that total cholesterol was lowered, risk of death from coronary heart disease would decrease by 15 percent. Also, they found that total mortality risk would drop by 11 percent.

The researchers concluded further that the reduction in deaths could be explained by the lipid-lowering ability of the statins. (See *Circulation,* vol. 97, 1998, pp. 946–52.)

Clearly, lowering cholesterol the natural way is preferable—but do bring those numbers down, even if you must take reduced drug doses.

8

The Best Medicine You Ever Ate

Larry is a British executive in his mid-forties. After buying a Benecol spread when it became available in the United Kingdom, he became curious about how the product might influence his lipid levels. So he decided to try a two-week supply of the spread.

Intent on being as "scientific" as possible, he first asked his doctor to order a blood test before he began to use the Benecol so that he could establish a clear baseline set of lipid measurements. He found that his total cholesterol was relatively low, at 167—a reading that placed him in the "low" risk category, as designated in chart 1 on page 30.

But Larry's "good" HDL cholesterol was also quite low, at 34—a level that placed him in the "high" risk category for cardiovascular disease.

As a result of these findings, Larry's physician calculated that his ratio of total cholesterol to HDL cholesterol was 4.91—a measurement that put him in the "borderline" category for that particular value. (To be "acceptable," his ratio should have been 3.5 to 4.2.)

Unfortunately, there was little prospect for Larry to

raise his HDL cholesterol through exercise. He was already quite athletic—a competitive distance runner who worked out regularly four to five days per week. Yet this aerobic activity had not caused his HDL to budge by even one point.

But with the Benecol spread, Larry now had another option. So he began to eat the recommended amounts— three pats per day, one at each meal—over a two-week period. The size of the servings was relatively small at 8 grams, but that was enough to cover a piece of bread or to melt on a piece of corn on the cob.

After two weeks, Larry asked to have his cholesterol level measured again—and he was shocked. His total cholesterol had dropped down to 139, even though his HDL had stayed almost the same, at 35. This meant that the functional food had lowered his ratio from that borderline 4.91 down to 3.97, a result that put him squarely in the "acceptable" risk category.

But there's more to Larry's story.

He was curious about what would happen if he went off the Benecol. So he stopped eating the spread for five days and had his blood tested once more. He found that his cholesterol had gone back up to the prenutriceutical level of 167.

I immediately saw that Larry was a classic case of how a margarine containing stanol esters from the rapeseed plant is supposed to work in the human system. The plant extract, taken in the recommended amounts per day, in effect seems to "bathe" the digestive tract with protection.

The plant stanols stand guard as cholesterol from the diet and from the circulating bile tries to reenter the bloodstream through the micelles. These, you'll recall, are the tiny, slippery containers that introduce cholesterol back into the bloodstream through the walls of the small intestine. The plant stanols in effect "boot" the cholesterol from the micelles—and may destroy the micelles as well.

But when the plant stanols are removed—as happened when Larry stopped eating the Benecol—the cholesterol reverts to its old tricks in the bloodstream. It's likely, in other words, that when you stop the nutriceutical, your cholesterol will rise to its original level.

Despite the promising results, it may take more for you to become enthusiastic about a new food product. You want to know: What does it cost, and how does it taste?

The Cost and Taste Tests

These lipid-controlling functional foods obviously have tremendous potential for your health—but are they within your family food budget? What can you expect to pay for them?

The short answer is that you'll pay several times more for a functional food than for a comparable product. Take Control, for instance, is currently selling at several times the price of an equivalent amount of margarine. But, of course, the cholesterol-lowering benefits of Take Control far surpass those of an ordinary spread—and the functional food costs much less than a prescription medication. As more products become available and the science of processing them advances, the costs will undoubtedly come down. But in the meantime, you should expect to pay more for a cholesterol-lowering nutriceutical spread, salad dressing, or yogurt than for a nonnutriceutical equivalent.

What about the flavor? My "taste testing" of the Benecol spread and two salad dressings (the thousand island and the ranch) as well as Take Control has confirmed for me that these products are comparable to more familiar margarine spreads and dressings. There's no aftertaste or other indication that you're eating a "de-signed" food. You'll find they fit easily into your daily food plan—and you may even like them better than the nonnutriceutical foods you're now eating. (The yogurt wasn't available for a taste test at the time this book went to press.)

In a few pages, I'll share some practical suggestions for meal preparation using specific functional foods. But before you begin your meal preparation, it's important to understand some simple points about these functional foods that will enable you to get the maximum health benefits, as well as the maximum taste effects.

First, we'll focus on meal-planning principles and guidelines that are related to the designed functional foods, such as Benecol and Take Control. Then, we'll consider some strategies for the traditional functional foods that contain soluble fiber.

A Game Plan for Getting the Most Out of Any Designed Functional Food

To maximize your health benefits from designed functional foods, keep these principles in mind as you stock up on the various products that appear on your supermarket shelves:

Principle 1: Follow the Instructions Exactly

Above all, this means consuming precisely the amounts recommended on the product label. Typically, you'll consume 3 pats (or small containers) of the spread per day, or 6 tablespoons of the salad dressings.

These servings are based on scientific research, which has shown that the average person will derive the greatest benefits from the amounts indicated. If you eat less than the recommended amount, you can expect that you will experience a smaller drop in your cholesterol. On the other hand, if you eat more than the recommended amount, it's uncertain that you will derive a greater benefit.

You should also divide your consumption over three meals, just as the instructions suggest. The idea is to keep your small intestines *bathed* with the plant extract, so that it can prevent the cholesterol from moving through the intestinal wall. If you try to consume your entire daily dose of the nutriceutical in the morning or in the evening, you won't be getting the complete "coverage" you need.

Remember: Cholesterol comes into your small intestines at various times during the day—either through your diet or through the circulation of bile from your liver.

Another important point to keep in mind is that the average person takes in about 400 mg of cholesterol per day through the diet, and even more, 1,000 mg per day, moves back into your blood through the circulation and the reabsorption process occurring in your small intestines. You have to have enough of the plant stanol extract present in your body to be able to "kick" that cholesterol out of those micelles. That's the only way you can hope to maximize the amount that will be washed away in your bowel movements.

Principle 2: Use Different Functional Foods During the Course of a Day

Most people become bored if they have to eat the same food day in and day out. Even spreads can begin to wear after a time. The antidote to this problem is to mix and mingle cholesterol-lowering nutriceutical products from meal to meal.

For example, you might like to put the spread on your

toast in the morning. But then you prefer the yogurt at lunch. Finally, it's natural to reach for the salad dressing in the evening. You can get exactly the same benefits from this sort of variety that you receive by sticking to one product.

Principle 3: Minimize Cooking with Products Containing Plant Stanol and Sterol Extracts— at Least for the Time Being

Some tests have suggested that the Benecol spread can withstand heat as high as 450 degrees Fahrenheit. McNeil representatives approve of the use of the regular Benecol spread for cooking. But Lipton representatives recommend against use of the Take Control spread in cooking. Melting the spreads over foods—such as hot baked potatoes—is fine, however.

There are also some other cooking concerns. If you heat the Benecol spread in a skillet or pan, or combine it with other ingredients for baking, you're sure to lose some of the plant stanol extract. Remember that your primary objective is to get the operative cholesterol-lowering components into your digestive tract!

In addition, it can be very expensive to use these nutriceutical spreads for cooking. Typically, to make muffins or cookies, for instance, you have to use much more, over and above the recommended daily dose of three pats.

On the other hand, if you're willing to spend the extra money, you may find that the cooking option can help maximize your ability to lower your total and "bad" LDL cholesterol. I've included several recipes and meal suggestions that include Benecol as an option in cooking. Amounts above the usual recommended daily doses have been suggested in the recipes because of the likelihood of losing some of the product in the cooking process.

Some Nutritional Rules for Soluble Fiber

To have the maximum effect, soluble-fiber products, including cereals, should be mixed with other foods as part of a meal—and not eaten between meals—according to researchers from the Department of Nutritional Sciences, Faculty of Medicine, St. Michael's Hospital, Toronto. (See *American Journal of Clinical Nutrition,* vol. 59, May 1994, pp. 1055–59.)

In this study, 18 participants with modestly high cholesterol levels consumed 7.3 grams per day of psyllium for two weeks through an enriched cereal. The results: Their total cholesterol dropped by 8 percent; their "bad" LDL cholesterol declined by 11 percent; and their "good" HDL cholesterol went down by 7 percent. But when the same cereal servings were eaten between meals, the participants' total, LDL, and HDL cholesterol were the same as those of the controls. In other words, the soluble fiber had no effect. A possible reason for this result is that the soluble fiber may bind the dietary cholesterol in other foods in the intestines and usher it out of the body before it can enter the bloodstream.

How much soluble fiber should you eat, and how often?

Nutritional experts recommend that the total daily dietary fiber intake for adults should be in the range of 20 to 35 grams per day—even though the average is about 14 to 15 grams per day. (See *American Journal of Medicine,* vol. 106, Jan. 25, 1999, pp. 46S–51S.)

Of this total, at least 8 to 10 grams per day, and preferably more, should come from soluble-fiber products, such as oat bran or psyllium, which have been scientifically proven to have the ability to lower cholesterol by 5 to 8 percent or even more in many people.

If you are able to consume more than 10 grams of soluble fiber per day, there is a chance you'll be able to lower your cholesterol by 10 percent or even more. If you haven't been eating much soluble fiber, the unanswered question is how well your blood lipids will respond to this functional food. The only way to find out is include some oats, psyllium, and rhubarb in your diet—and that's what the following recipe and meal suggestion sections are all about.

In the first section, you'll be given recipes and suggestions that related to the designed functional foods, such as Benecol. In the second section, we'll turn to the traditional functional foods, which mainly operate through soluble fiber.

Recipes and Meal Suggestions for Designed Functional Foods

Starting with a Spread

The time has arrived to take charge of your cholesterol right at your own kitchen table—and we'll begin with the margarinelike spreads.

The basic strategy is to divide your daily "dose" into 3 servings (3 8-gram containers) per day with meals or snacks. You might choose the regular Benecol spread, which contains 45 calories per serving, or the "light" spread, which has only 30 calories per serving. Lipton recommends 1 to 2 servings (1 to 2 tablespoons) per day of Take Control, which contains 50 calories per serving.

There are some tried-and-true ways to make the most efficient and simplest use of these spreads (with minimal loss of those potent plant stanol esters!):

- **For breakfast:** Put your spread on low-fat or no-fat muffins; bagels; whole wheat or whole grain toast; pancakes; waffles; or oatmeal (a combination that will give you a double functional food wallop, with Benecol or Take Control plus a soluble-fiber food).

- **For lunch or snack:** Apply the spread to rolls and bread; reduced-fat or no-fat crackers; pretzels; or sandwiches.

- **For the evening meal:** Use the nutriceutical spread on rolls and bread; reduced-fat or no-fat crackers (as with an appetizer or soup); rice; pasta; baked potatoes; baked sweet potatoes; hot vegetables; or fish.

Using such easy yet effective techniques, a plant extract spread such as the Benecol or Take Control product can do a great job of livening up the taste of common foods and snacks. In fact, if you are particularly conscientious about your diet, you may do your best to avoid before-meal spreads as an appetizer. But now you have an option that allows you to lower your cholesterol and enjoy that appetizer guilt-free. An added benefit, by the way, is that both the Take Control and Benecol spreads are relatively high in monounsaturated fat, which helps lower cholesterol, and low in saturated fat, which raises cholesterol.

Now let's consider some meal tips that are a little fancier.

You'll still find these suggestions easy to prepare and employ with your personal food plans. By following these simple tips, you can create something different with Benecol or other functional food spreads every day of the week.

(Although the basic ideas for these meal tips were developed for Benecol products by Kitchen Consultants, National Network Creative Solutions, their original versions have been edited and expanded with nutritional information from other sources.)

....

Breakfast Spreads

1. Top 1 serving of cooked oatmeal or other hot cereal with 1 serving of Benecol regular or light spread.

2. Spread 1 serving of Benecol light spread over 1 serving of toasted, reduced-fat waffles.

3. For a no-cholesterol egg dish with "punch," melt 1 serving of Benecol regular spread, and pour it over 3 scrambled egg whites or scrambled egg substitute. Top the entire dish off with salsa.

4. Steam 1 cup of sliced apples until they are tender. Transfer the apples to a bowl. Immediately use a knife to cover the hot apples with 1 serving of Benecol regular spread. As the spread melts, sprinkle the entire dish with cinnamon and a pinch or two of sugar.

5. Melt 1 serving of Benecol regular spread over 2 cups hot diced red potatoes, chopped onions, and bell peppers, for a healthy breakfast combination.

6. Melt 1 serving of Benecol regular spread over 1 cup of hot hash browns.

7. Mix 1 or 2 tablespoons of your favorite reduced-calorie fruit spread with 1 serving of Benecol light spread. Serve over 2 slices of toast.

8. Prepare a zesty orange spread by combining 1 serving of Benecol regular or light spread with minced orange peels and a little orange juice. Serve over 2 slices of toast, 2 biscuits, or 2 English muffin halves.

9. Prepare an almond spread for 2 muffins by mixing 1 serving of Benecol regular spread with finely chopped almonds and a hint of almond extract.

....
....

Lunch Spreads

1. Stir ⅛ cup of chopped sun-dried tomatoes into 1 serving of Benecol regular or light spread. Use this mixture instead of mayonnaise on bread (2 slices) when making a sandwich.

2. To add a sweet topping to 1 large piece of cornbread, stir 2 tablespoons of honey into 1 serving of Benecol regular or light spread. Cover the top surface of the cornbread with the mixture.

3. Make a regular or light garlic spread (2 teaspoons) by stirring a finely chopped fresh garlic clove into 1 serving of Benecol regular or light spread. If you want to make a larger amount, keep the unused portion on hand in the refrigerator. Use it later to make garlic toast or to provide a final garnish to poultry, fish, mushrooms, or green beans.

4. Make 2 slices of Parmesan cheese toast by spreading

thinly sliced French bread with 1 serving of Benecol regular spread. Then sprinkle with grated Parmesan cheese. Broil the bread until golden, or toasted to taste. Serve with salad.

5. Benecol-broiled peaches (2 halves) make a great addition to a simple salad lunch. Spread 1 serving of Benecol regular spread on cut, "scooped" sides of fresh pitted or canned peaches. (The spread should be placed in the pitted cavity of the peach half.) Broil until golden.

6. Dress up salads with the added flavor and crunch of toasted nuts. Heat 1 serving of regular Benecol spread with $1/2$ cup walnuts, pecans, almonds, or pine nuts in a skillet. Stir until golden. (Some of the spread will be lost in this process, so you may want to use a double serving.)

7. Make Italian bread sticks (2 sticks) by spreading rolled-out refrigerated pizza dough with 1 serving of Benecol regular spread. Top with an Italian herb seasoning and grated Parmesan cheese. Cut the dough into strips, and bake them until golden. Serve with pasta salad. (This has been designed as a serving for one person.)

8. Tarragon-mustard topping adds great taste with little effort to grilled chicken (1 piece) or freshly steamed rice (1 cup). Stir small amounts of chopped fresh or dried tarragon and Dijon mustard into 1 serving of Benecol regular spread. Add it to the chicken or rice just after it has been cooked and immediately before serving.

9. Mix 1 serving of Benecol regular spread with a sprinkling of fresh or dried dill weed. Pour over 1 cup mixed steamed carrots, green beans, and broccoli.

10. Add a little excitement to a baked potato (1 potato) by stirring 1 teaspoon sliced fresh or dried chives into 1 serving of Benecol regular spread. Use it as a topping over the potato.

Supper Spreads

1. Sprinkle extra flavor and crunch over 1 cup of simple steamed vegetables or a casserole with this topping: Stir ¼ cup seasoned breadcrumbs into 1 serving of Benecol regular or light spread.

2. Jazz up 1 cup of steamed green beans by drizzling a mixture of 1 serving of melted Benecol regular spread, a touch of lemon juice, and salt and pepper to taste over the top.

3. Moisten corn on the cob (1 piece) with 1 serving of Benecol regular or light spread. To enhance the flavor, sprinkle the spread with Italian herb blend, salt, and pepper before applying it to the corn.

4. Try this garlic-crumb-coated pasta dish: Combine 1 teaspoon minced garlic with 1 serving of Benecol regular spread. Then stir in ⅓ cup seasoned breadcrumbs. Sprinkle the mixture over 1½ cups of hot, cooked tube-shaped pasta.

5. Add excitement to a simple pan-fried or grilled burger (1 patty) by adding a southwestern topping: Stir a teaspoon of chili powder and garlic salt into 1 serving of Benecol regular or light spread. Allow the mixture to melt over the warm hamburger just before serving.

6. Add a Mediterranean flavoring to grilled or broiled chicken breasts with this combination: Mix 1 serving of Benecol regular or light spread, ½ teaspoon garlic salt, and ½ teaspoon dried herb seasoning. Then spread over 1 warm chicken breast.

7. Chili-lime spread is great when melted over 1 serving of cooked scallops, shrimp, or chicken. Mix 1 tablespoon lime juice and chili powder with 1 serving of Benecol regular spread.

8. Baked onions are a delicious side dish. Cut both ends off 1 medium-sized onion and peel. Make three or four deep cuts in the onion at different points. Mix a sprinkling of fresh or dried oregano, salt and pepper to taste, and 2 servings of Benecol regular spread. Spread the mixture over the onion and inside the cut portions. Wrap in foil and bake for about 1½ hours, or until tender. Pour any remaining juices over the onion before serving.

9. Create an Asian topping for 1 piece of grilled or broiled chicken or fish: Beat 1 tablespoon each of soy sauce, ground ginger, and garlic powder into 1 serving of Benecol regular or light spread. Place the mixture over warm poultry or fish, and allow it to melt before serving.

10. For a simple pasta primavera, melt 1 serving of Benecol regular spread in a skillet, and add 1 cup chopped broccoli, zucchini, carrots, and mushrooms. Cook until "crunchy" to taste. Pour into a bowl with 1½ cups of hot pasta, and toss.

Spreads for Snacks

1. Prepare tasty and healthy popcorn by drizzling 2 servings of melted Benecol regular spread over 3 cups of air-popped popcorn. The best time to do the drizzling is in the last few seconds of popping. Then mix up the popped popcorn one more time by hand and serve.

2. Make a sweet snack by brushing 2 servings of Benecol regular spread on top of 2 soft bread sticks. Sprinkle with cinnamon sugar, and bake until warm and soft.

3. Prepare quesadillas by melting 1 serving of Benecol spread in a skillet. Put 1 or 2 flour tortillas (depending on your appetite and the size of the tortillas) in the skillet. Cover the tortillas with 1 additional serving of Benecol, and also spread on your favorite cheese and a chopped-up vegetable (like broccoli or red peppers). Heat until the cheese is melted and serve.

4. Serve crostini (2 pieces) by spreading 1 serving of Benecol regular spread on each side of a single serving of sliced French bread (baguette). Top with fresh chopped tomatoes and basil. Sprinkle lightly with shredded Parmesan or mozzarella cheese, if desired. Broil until warm and toasted.

5. Prepare tortilla chips (two 6-to-8-inch tortillas) by spreading 2 servings of Benecol regular spread over corn or flour tortillas. Cut them into wedges, and bake until light brown and crisp.

....

The Dressing Alternative

Spreads start out as the basic designed functional food for lowering cholesterol, but other products are not far behind. One of these is a staple of many of our meals, especially at lunch and dinnertime—salad dressing.

In this section, I've included a number of suggestions about how to use the Benecol dressings at each meal. But remember: If you choose to substitute another, comparable cholesterol-lowering nutriceutical for a particular meal—such as a spread for breakfast—that's perfectly all right. In fact, the variety may even be advisable to help you avoid boredom and stick with your functional food strategy.

(Again, these meal suggestions have been developed originally by Kitchen Consultants, National Network Creative Solutions, for special use with Benecol salad dressings. The instructions have been revised, edited, and adapted to fit the special needs of this book.)

Breakfast Dressings

1. Make a bagel spread by mixing fat-free cream cheese with 1 serving (2 tablespoons) Benecol Ranch Dressing, sliced green onions, and chopped smoked salmon. Spread over 2 toasted bagel halves.

2. Enjoy a fruit dip by combining 1 serving (2 tablespoons) Benecol French Dressing with 2½ tablespoons honey and poppy seeds. Serve with fresh-cut fruit, such as apples, pears, berries, peaches, and bananas.

3. Mix 1 serving (2 tablespoons) of your favorite Benecol dressing into ¼ cup fat-free cream cheese. Spread on bagel chips, crackers, or rice cakes.

4. Dip freshly washed and chilled grapes into 1 serving (2 tablespoons) Benecol Ranch Dressing. (To avoid wasting any of the functional food, mop up the remainder with a piece of toast.)

5. Give cottage cheese (½ to 1 cup, according to your appetite) more excitement by stirring in 1 serving (2 tablespoons) Benecol French or Thousand Island Dressing. Serve with sliced fruit on the side.

Lunch Dressings

1. For one pita pocket sandwich, stir dill weed into 1 serving (2 tablespoons) Benecol Ranch Dressing. Stuff the pita pockets with lean roast beef, chopped tomatoes, and sliced cucumbers. Pour the dressing inside.

2. Give three-bean salad a new twist by marinating 1 cup of your favorite beans in 1 serving (2 tablespoons) Benecol Creamy Italian Dressing.

3. For an open-faced turkey sandwich, spread 2 toasted French bread slices with 1 serving (2 tablespoons)

Benecol French Dressing. Top with roasted turkey slices and cranberry sauce.

4. Use 1 serving (2 tablespoons) Benecol Ranch or Creamy Italian Dressing when making 1 cup coleslaw. Add a sprinkling of celery seed.

5. Substitute your favorite Benecol Dressing for mayonnaise on all types of sandwiches.

Dinner Dressings

1. For marinated vegetables with pizzazz: Toss 1 serving (2 tablespoons) Benecol Ranch or Creamy Italian Dressing with 1 cup of a combination of cooled steamed vegetables—like carrots, green beans, peas, broccoli, and cauliflower. Chill for about 1 hour to allow the flavors to develop.

2. Make an Italian pasta salad by pouring 1 serving (2 tablespoons) Benecol Creamy Italian Dressing over 1 cup of your favorite cold or hot pasta, mozzarella cheese, and vegetables.

3. Serve a dish with Asian flair by mixing 1 serving (2 tablespoons) Benecol Creamy Italian dressing with a little soy sauce, ground or fresh ginger, sliced green onions, and chopped fresh cilantro. Serve over snow pea pods, mushrooms, crisp Chinese noodles, or chicken tenders and rice.

4. For added color and flavor in your macaroni or potato salad (1 cup), mix in 1 serving (2 tablespoons) Benecol French or Thousand Island Dressing instead of mayonnaise.

5. Drizzle 1 serving (2 tablespoons) of your favorite Benecol dressing over strips of grilled chicken (1 cup). Serve with melon slices on a bed of lettuce.

Dressings for Snacks

1. Make a serving of lemon-chive dip by mixing 1 serving (2 tablespoons) Benecol Ranch Dressing with 2 tablespoons lemon juice, lemon peel, and fresh or dried sliced chives. Serve in a small dip dish for use with vegetables or crackers. (To get the full benefits of the nutriceutical, be sure to use all of the dip.)

2. For a dip, spread, or dressing with extra punch: Stir 3 tablespoons of prepared salsa or picante sauce into 1 serving (2 tablespoons) Benecol Thousand Island Dressing.

3. Make a spinach dip by mixing 1 serving (2 tablespoons) Benecol Creamy Italian Dressing with $\frac{1}{4}$ cup fat-free sour cream and 1 box of thawed well-drained frozen chopped spinach and sliced green onions. Dip pretzels or veggies.

4. Prepare a dill dip by mixing $\frac{1}{4}$ cup fat-free mayonnaise with 1 serving (2 tablespoons) Benecol French Style Dressing. Add fresh or dried dill weed. Serve with fresh-cut vegetables such as carrots, cucumbers, mushrooms, celery, asparagus, snow pea pods, or endive spears.

5. Make a Dijon dip by mixing 1 serving (2 tablespoons) of Benecol Thousand Island Dressing with $2\frac{1}{2}$ tablespoons Dijon-style mustard. Serve with fresh vegetables, bread sticks, or pretzels.

Recipes and Meal
Suggestions for Traditional
Functional Foods

In this section, we are going to focus on recipes that contain traditional functional foods, such as oats, psyllium, and other grain-based products. There are a number of cereal brands and other food products, produced by companies such as Quaker Oats, which contain soluble fiber that has been associated with lower cholesterol. In any event, I'd suggest that you focus mainly on those containing high amounts of oat bran and psyllium.

Many of the suggestions on preparing psyllium dishes come from the Kellogg Company, whose Ensemble line features functional foods that lower cholesterol, mainly through the bile-binding action of soluble fiber. Kellogg also has produced a number of frozen and other commercially prepared foods that include significant amounts of psyllium in the ingredients. These products are relatively low in fat, with fewer than 30 percent of total calories—and often much less—derived from fat. Also, many carry 2 to 4 grams of soluble fiber per serving, with much of that coming from psyllium.

Remember: If you take in at least about 8 grams of soluble fiber per day, you'll have a good chance to begin to get significant cholesterol-lowering action—provided your body chemistry is the type that responds well to the bile-binding mechanism.

The particular Kellogg products that appear to have the most value as low-fat, cholesterol-lowering functional foods include: Kellogg's All-Bran Bran Buds, Apple Cinnamon Cereal, Honey-Nut Cereal (with Almonds), Multi-Grain Cereal, and Split-Top Stone Ground Wheat Bread.

The Bran Buds cereal contains 4 grams of soluble fiber per serving, with a significant portion of that coming from psyllium-seed husks. Each of the other products contains 3 grams of soluble fiber.

Some of the products that have 2 grams of soluble fiber per serving are Linguini Marinara Frozen Entrée,

Cheese Ravioli in Marinara Sauce, and Fettucini Alfredo Frozen Entrée.

Although only one serving of 2 grams per day is not really adequate to have an impact on lowering your cholesterol, it's a start. And of course, you can add additional servings at other meals. Or you might boost your daily "dose" significantly by combining a Kellogg product with additional vegetables and grains that contain soluble fiber, such as oats or rhubarb.

In this traditional functional food section, I've also included recipes using oat bran and rhubarb. As we saw in chapter 6, both of these foods have significant power to lower blood cholesterol through the soluble-fiber mechanism.

....

Bran Buds Muffins

Ingredients

1½ cups Kellogg's Bran Buds with psyllium cereal
1¼ cups all-purpose flour
½ cup sugar
¼ teaspoon salt
1 tablespoon baking powder
1¼ cups skim milk
1 egg or 2 egg whites
¼ cup vegetable oil

Instructions

1. In an electric blender or food processor, crush the Bran Buds cereal to fine crumbs.
2. Stir together crushed cereal, flour, sugar, salt, and baking powder. Set aside.
3. In a large mixing bowl, combine the milk, egg, and

oil. Mix well. Add flour mixture, stirring only until combined. Portion the batter evenly into twelve lightly greased 2½-inch muffin pan cups.

4. Bake at 400°F about 20 minutes or until golden brown. Serve warm.

Yield *12 muffins*

Nutritional Information (1 muffin) Calories—160, total fat—6 gm, saturated fat—1 gm, cholesterol—25 mg, dietary fiber—4 gm, sodium—215 mg.

....

....

Frosted Spice Cookies

Ingredients for the cookies

  1 *cup Kellogg's Bran Buds cereal*
 ½ *cup skim milk*
1½ *cups all-purpose flour*
 ½ *teaspoon baking soda*
 ½ *teaspoon cinnamon*
 ¼ *teaspoon nutmeg*
 ¼ *teaspoon ginger*
  1 *cup firmly packed brown sugar*
 ½ *cup regular margarine, softened, or Benecol margarine*
  3 *egg whites*
  1 *teaspoon vanilla*
  1 *cup raisins*
 ¼ *cup chopped almonds*

Ingredients for the frosting

1¼ *cups confectioners' sugar*
  1 *teaspoon vanilla*

  2 *tablespoons skim milk*
  2 *tablespoons chopped almonds*

Instructions

1. Measure the Bran Buds cereal and the ½ cup milk
into a small mixing bowl. Combine. Let stand about 5
minutes or until the cereal absorbs the milk.
2. Stir together the flour, baking soda, and spices. Set
aside.
3. In a large mixing bowl, beat the brown sugar and
margarine until light and fluffy. Add the egg whites, the
1 teaspoon vanilla, and the cereal mixture. Beat well.
Mix in the dry ingredients, raisins, and the ¼ cup
almonds. Drop the mixture by tablespoons onto very
lightly greased baking sheets.
4. Bake at 375°F for about 11 minutes or until golden
brown. Remove from baking sheets and place on wire
racks. Frost while warm by combining the confectioners' sugar, vanilla, and milk. Sprinkle with almonds. Let
stand until cool and the frosting is set before storing in
airtight container.

Yield 4 dozen cookies

Nutritional Information (2 cookies) Calories—160,
total fat—5 gm, saturated fat—1 gm, cholesterol—0 mg,
dietary fiber—2 gm.

....
....

Sweet Spoon-On

Ingredients

  2 *tablespoons warm water*
  ¼ *cup honey*

½ teaspoon ground cinnamon
2 cups Kellogg's Bran Buds cereal

Instructions

1. Blend together the water, honey, and cinnamon. Pour over the Bran Buds cereal in a large bowl. Immediately toss to moisten.

2. Gently spread on a lightly oiled baking sheet. Bake at 325°F for about 15 to 20 minutes until dry and crisp. Cool completely. Store in an airtight container.

Yield About 2 cups

Nutritional Information (1 tablespoon) Calories— 20, dietary fiber—1.5 gm, fat—between 0 and 1 gm.

Suggested Uses Sprinkle on cereal, yogurt, fresh fruit, stewed fruit, or cottage cheese. Use as a baking ingredient.

Variation After 10 minutes of baking time, sprinkle 2 teaspoons grated orange or lemon peel over the mixture. Stir gently. Continue baking about 10 minutes longer, as directed above.

··

Savory Spoon-On

Ingredients

2 tablespoons Worcestershire sauce
1 tablespoon lemon juice
½ teaspoon hot pepper sauce
2 cups Kellogg's Bran Buds cereal

Instructions

1. Mix Worcestershire sauce, lemon juice, and hot pep-

per sauce to blend thoroughly. Pour over Bran Buds
cereal in a large bowl. Immediately toss to moisten
evenly.
2. Spread evenly on a lightly oiled baking sheet.
3. Bake at 325°F for about 12 to 15 minutes, until dry
and crisp.

Yield About 2 cups

Nutritional Information (1 tablespoon) Calories—
15, dietary fiber—1.5 gm, fat—1 gm.

Suggested Uses Sprinkle on baked potatoes, hot
cooked vegetables, salads, and cottage cheese. Mix into
dips and meat loaves.

....

....

Fiber-Rich Mix

Ingredients

  2 *cups Kellogg's Bran Buds cereal*
  2 *cups Kellogg's Bran Flakes cereal*
  1 *cup sliced almonds, dried, unsalted*
  1/2 *cup raisins*
  1/2 *cup chopped* dried *apricots*
  1/2 *cup pitted prunes*

Instructions

1. Mix the two cereals. Then in a separate bowl combine the almonds and dried fruits separately.
2. Store the two mixes separately in tightly covered
containers or plastic food bags.
3. For one dry serving, combine 1/2 cup cereal mixture
with 1/3 cup nut-fruit mixture.

4. For one breakfast cereal serving, add skim milk to one mix serving.

Yield 8 servings

Nutritional Information (1 serving) Calories—260, Dietary fiber—11.7 gm.

One serving includes about ⅓ cup of Bran Buds, which contains 4 gm soluble fiber from psyllium husks. Each serving contains about 80 fat calories, or approximately 30 percent of total calories in each serving. Most of these fat calories come from the almonds.

Date Pie Crust

Ingredients

1 cup Kellogg's Bran Buds cereal
½ cup pitted dates
¾ cup all-purpose flour
2 tablespoons firmly packed brown sugar
¼ cup margarine (regular or Benecol)
2 tablespoons cold water

Instructions

1. Place Bran Buds cereal, dates, flour, sugar, and margarine in a food processor container. Process for about 30 seconds or until evenly combined and the dates are finely chopped. Add water, mixing until the mixture clumps together. Press the mixture firmly into the bottom and onto the sides of a 9-inch pie pan.
2. Bake at 400°F for about 10 minutes or until lightly browned. Cool completely. Note: The pie crust can

be cooked in a microwave oven on "high" for 90 seconds.

Yield One 9-inch pie crust

Nutritional Information ($^1/_8$ pie crust) Calories—169, dietary fiber—4 gm, fat—5.9 gm with regular margarine (32% of total serving calories), *or* fat—5.2 gm with Benecol regular spread (27.7% of total serving calories).

....
....

Old-Fashioned Oatmeal Banana Pancakes

Ingredients

$1^1/_2$ cups uncooked oatmeal
2 cups buttermilk
2 egg whites
1 cup whole wheat flour
2 teaspoons baking soda
1 mashed banana

Instructions

1. Mix the oatmeal, buttermilk, and egg whites. Let the mixture stand for at least $^1/_2$ hour, or refrigerate up to 24 hours.
2. Add the remaining ingredients, and stir the batter until the dry ingredients are moist.
3. Ladle about $^1/_4$ cup of batter onto a hot, lightly oiled griddle or frying pan.
4. Cook until lightly browned on both sides.

Yield 12 pancakes (diameter = 5 inches)

One Serving 2 pancakes

Nutritional Information (1 pancake) Calories—98, fat—1 gm, cholesterol—1 mg, fiber (soluble)—1 gm.

Raisin Oat-Bran Muffins

Ingredients

$1^{1}/_{4}$ cups oat-bran cereal
  1 cup whole wheat flour
$^{1}/_{3}$ cup raisins
  1 tablespoon baking power
$^{1}/_{2}$ cup skim milk
$^{1}/_{2}$ cup unsweetened orange juice
$^{1}/_{4}$ cup honey
  2 tablespoons safflower oil
  3 egg whites

Instructions

1. Preheat oven to 425°F.
2. Combine the dry ingredients.
3. To this mixture, add the skim milk, orange juice, honey, oil, and egg whites. Mix thoroughly.
4. Spread the mixture evenly among 12 regular-sized muffin tins.
5. Bake for about 20 minutes, or until lightly browned.

Yield 12 muffins

One Serving 2 muffins

Nutritional Information (1 muffin) Calories—132, cholesterol—0 mg, fat—1 gm, fiber (soluble)—1 gm.

Oatmeal Raisin Cookies

Ingredients

  1 cup whole wheat flour, sifted
 $1/2$ teaspoon baking soda
 $1/2$ teaspoon salt
 $1/4$ teaspoon ground cinnamon
 $1/8$ teaspoon nutmeg
$1^1/2$ cups quick-cooking oats
  2 egg whites, slightly beaten
 $1/4$ cup brown sugar
 $1/4$ cup chopped dates
 $1/3$ cup oil
 $1/2$ cup skim milk
  1 teaspoon vanilla extract
  1 cup raisins

Instructions

1. Preheat oven to 375°F.
2. Using a bowl, combine the flour, baking soda, salt, cinnamon, and nutmeg. Stir in the oats.
3. Using a second bowl, mix together the egg whites, brown sugar, dates, oil, skim milk, vanilla, and raisins. Add this mixture to the flour mixture, and mix all thoroughly.
4. Drop this batter onto an oiled cookie sheet, one teaspoon at a time.
5. Bake 12–15 minutes, depending on the texture you prefer. A shorter baking time will result in a chewy, soft cookie, while longer baking will produce a crisper cookie.

Yield   24 cookies

One Serving 2 cookies

Nutritional Information (1 cookie) Calories—100, fat—3 gm, cholesterol—0 mg, fiber (soluble)—1 gm.

....

....

Strawberry Rhubarb

Ingredients

1 *pound rhubarb stalks, leaves removed*
$1/2$ *cup nonfat, low-calorie seedless strawberry jam*
$1/2$ *teaspoon powdered ginger*

Instructions

1. Cut the rhubarb stalks into thin strips. Then cut the strips into one-inch lengths.
2. Preheat oven to 350°F.
3. Apply a thin coating of the jam to the bottom of a relatively small baking tin.
4. Sprinkle the ginger over the remainder of the jam.
5. Coat the cut rhubarb with the jam-ginger mix, then spread the rhubarb strips evenly across the bottom of the tin.
6. Bake for 30–40 minutes, depending on how soft you prefer the rhubarb.

Yield 6 equal servings

Nutritional Information (per 3-ounce serving) Calories—150, fat—0 gm, cholesterol—0 mg, fiber (soluble)—4 gm.

....

9

Women and Cholesterol

Can functional foods help women with heart disease?

Let's take a look at the results of a 1997 Finnish study that involved 32 postmenopausal women, ranging in age from 48 to 56. All of them had suffered a previous myocardial infarction, or heart attack.

Doctors Helena Gylling and Tatu A. Miettinen— University of Helsinki scientists who have broken much new ground in plant stanol research—conducted their investigation by testing in various ways the effect on the women of a rapeseed (canola) oil margarine that contains a plant stanol ester. (See *Circulation,* vol. 96, Dec. 16, 1997, pp. 4226–31.)

In one part of the double-blind study, a group of the women, who were not on cholesterol-lowering medications, ate servings of the plant stanol margarine for seven weeks. Their total daily servings included 3 grams of the plant extract. As a result of the biological action of the designed functional food, this group lowered their total cholesterol by 13 percent and their "bad" LDL cholesterol by 20 percent.

Another group took *both* the cholesterol-lowering

medication simvastatin (Zocor) *and* the plant stanol margarine for a 12-week period. The researchers found that on top of significant lipid reductions through the drug, the plant stanol margarine caused *additional* declines of 11 percent in total cholesterol and 16 percent in LDL cholesterol!

The scientists determined that using the plant stanol functional food alone produced normal total and LDL measurements in one-third of the women (all of whom had suffered a previous heart attack). Also, the researchers found that the functional food could *replace* the simvastatin drug in a significant number of the women and *reduce* the drug dose in many of the remaining cases.

In effect, then, this study demonstrates an important way that the Compound Effect can work for female heart patients, as the functional food is added to—or in some cases, substituted for—the cholesterol-lowering drug.

These and other studies have demonstrated that designed functional foods, such as Benecol, seem to work as well for women as for men. But how do women respond to the traditional functional foods, such as those that operate in the body through the action of soluble fiber?

Women and Traditional Functional Foods

Again, these foods appear to work as well for women as for men—according to a 1994 study on psyllium, conducted by the Department of Nutritional Sciences, Faculty of Medicine, University of Toronto in Ontario.

In that investigation, which was reported in the *American Journal of Clinical Nutrition* (vol. 307, April 1994, pp. 269–73), scientists evaluated 21 men and 21 women with high blood lipids, including high cholesterol. The participants all went on a low-fat NCEP diet (known as the Step II diet—see page 39). Also, they ate one of two types of cereal, the first containing 6.7 grams of psyllium fiber per day, and the second containing wheat bran.

At the end of two weeks, the psyllium cereals on average reduced total cholesterol by 6.4 percent and "bad" LDL cholesterol by 7.8 percent. Also, there was a modest drop in "good" HDL cholesterol—a normal result when total cholesterol is lowered significantly. Interestingly, the researchers found that the women tended to have greater decreases in all types of cholesterol from the psyllium than did the men.

Clearly, then, all types of functional foods can benefit women. Furthermore, the incentive to incorporate these new products into their cholesterol-fighting programs may intensify as women begin to focus more on their cardiovascular health.

Using Functional Foods to Meet a Woman's Special Needs

Although much research on cholesterol and cardiovascular disease has been done on men, it's only in recent years that investigators have explored some of the special concerns of women. Indeed, women are relative latecomers to the heart disease and cholesterol story.

In fact, an April 23, 1997, *JAMA* report revealed that less than one of every ten female heart patients had been given adequate treatment to bring their "bad" LDL cholesterol to safe levels. (See *JAMA,* vol. 277, no. 16, April 23–30, 1997, pp. 1281–86.)

The researchers said that even though half of the more than 2,700 women in the study were on lipid-lowering medications, 91 percent had failed to lower their LDL levels below the target threshold of 100, which is the goal many experts now set for patients with heart disease. (See chart 2 on page 31.)

Furthermore, nearly two-thirds of the women studied failed to lower their LDL below 130—which was an earlier goal established by the National Cholesterol Education Program Adult Treatment Panel. As you can see from the charts on pages 30 and 31, this means that the two-thirds at this LDL level who were *without* heart disease were in a "borderline" risk category. And those *with* heart or vessel disease, whose LDL readings were 130 or above, were at a "high" risk level.

An editorial that accompanied this study said that the failure to treat women properly and effectively for high or unbalanced cholesterol is based on two fallacious assumptions by many scientists and physicians.

First, some doctors believe incorrectly that women are at lower risk than men for heart disease because they forget that the extra protection women enjoy before menopause evaporates after menopause. Second, a few actually assume—despite the overwhelming weight of the evidence—that if women do receive medications, their bodies will be less responsive to treatment than those of men.

It is of course well known that before menopause, most women do enjoy more cardiovascular protection. The estrogen in their bodies keeps their "good" HDL cholesterol high, their total and "bad" LDL cholesterol relatively low, and their ratio of total to HDL cholesterol much lower than that of men.

With the onset of menopause, however, estrogen levels decrease, and women become as vulnerable as men to heart disease caused by blood-lipid imbalances. In fact, women may become *more* vulnerable as they grow older because they may fail to realize that the physical and hormonal changes that occurred at menopause have put them at serious risk.

It's at this point that functional foods can be of special help.

Controlling Cholesterol in a Grandmother

Jane, a 66-year-old specialty shop owner and grandmother, is part of a group that has sparked increasing concern among health professionals: postmenopausal women whose cholesterol has gone out of the control.

Before she went through menopause in her early fifties, Jane's cholesterol was normal. But her total cholesterol at her last blood test was 280, a figure that put her well up into the "high" risk category. (See chart 1 on page 30.) As for her "bad" LDL cholesterol, that measurement was 183—again, a result that put her in a "high" risk category.

Jane had other lipid problems as well. Her "good" HDL cholesterol was extremely low at 31—a reading that put her solidly in the "high" risk range. Also, the low HDL coupled with the high total cholesterol gave her a terrible total-to-HDL ratio of 9.03. This reading in effect placed her off the chart as a person at high risk for cardiovascular disease.

One of the first steps Jane took to get her cholesterol under control was to make use of a functional food. She ate recommended amounts of a Benecol margarine spread for an eight-week trial period—and found that her blood-lipid profile changed significantly for the better after only about three weeks.

As a result of the plant stanol spread, Jane's total cholesterol dropped to 242, which was still not ideal but was considerably healthier than 280. Also, this improvement placed her close to the "borderline" risk category. This decline represented a reduction of 13.6 percent in her total cholesterol.

Her "good" HDL cholesterol actually increased from

31 to 34—a rise of 9.7 percent. Also, her "bad" LDL went down from 183 to 163, or nearly 11 percent. Jane's triglyceride reading even declined by nearly 100 points to 238—even though these designed functional foods don't usually affect triglycerides.

At the end of the eight-week period, Jane found that her ratio had dropped from the alarmingly high reading of 9.03 to 7.21—an improvement of more than 20 percent.

It's true that this new ratio still placed her at high risk for cardiovascular disease. But at least she was now in a stronger position to take advantage of other natural cholesterol-lowering techniques—such as a low-fat diet, exercise, or a soluble-fiber functional food like psyllium. If pursued together, these had the potential to improve her cholesterol profile exponentially through the Compound Effect.

Despite such success stories, the diagnosis and treatment of heart and vessel problems in women continues to lag. And as more research emerges on women and cardiovascular disease, we are beginning to understand what a complex issue this is, for older women in particular.

What's So Special About a Woman's Heart?

Most of the special features of a woman's heart and cardiovascular system are related in some way to the event of menopause. This "change of life," which may unfold over a period of months or even years, is accompanied by a cessation of the menstrual cycle and a precipitous decline in the production of the female hormone estrogen.

Some of the most significant secondary physiological changes that accompany menopause involve imbalances in cholesterol and other blood lipids that have some connection to heart disease and cardiovascular risk. Here are some of the problems that may develop—and what can be done about them.

Problem: High "bad" LDL cholesterol and low "good" HDL cholesterol after menopause.

Solution for Women: Possible hormone replacement therapy (HRT), which includes a combination of the hormones estrogen and progestin.

Low doses of progestin with estrogen can significantly improve the balance of lipoprotein lipids (fats) in the blood of postmenopausal women. In particular, progestin can raise "good" HDL levels and reduce the ratio of total to HDL cholesterol. (See *American Journal of Obstetrics and Gynecology,* April 1998, pp. 787–92.)

Other studies have shown that hormone replacement therapy (HRT) can lower levels of "bad" LDL cholesterol by 15 percent and may raise "good" HDL by 15 to 30 percent. (See *Bottom Line Health,* vol. 12, no. 5, May 1998, pp. 1–3; *Women's Health Advisor,* vol. 2, no. 4, April 1998, pp. 1–3.)

Because there is some worry about an increased danger of breast cancer with estrogen, women who believe they are at risk for cancer may want to consider an alternative treatment such as raloxifene (Evista). This estrogenlike medication, sometimes known as a "designer estrogen," can lower LDL cholesterol without raising the risk for cancer.

The importance of estrogen has been emphasized in recent studies that show it can inhibit the susceptibility of "bad" LDL to become oxidized and can also reduce levels of LDL and increase the amounts of "good" HDL. (See *Maturitas,* Jan. 1998, pp. 229–34.)

The process of oxidation of LDL in the bloodstream

involves the ability of unstable oxygen molecules, or free radicals, to turn the LDL molecules into blobs of fat that stick to vessel walls. Many scientists regard this action as a key step in the formation of plaque in blood vessels and the development of atherosclerosis, which results in heart attacks and strokes. (For more on this topic—and how antioxidant supplements can be employed to combat oxidation—see Chapter 11.)

A caveat on estrogen: Some recent research findings suggest that even though HRT may be fine for women *without* a history of heart disease, women *with* heart disease may want to avoid this therapy. (See "Some Qualifications on Estrogen," page 178.)

Problem: Low levels of "good" HDL cholesterol. (Low HDLs are associated with higher risk of cardiovascular disease, while high HDLs are linked to lower risk.)

Solution for Women: Endurance exercise.

Exercise of moderate duration by aerobically fit premenopausal women, who ran on a treadmill 24 to 48 km (15 to 30 miles) per week, resulted in postexercise increases of HDL similar to those experienced by men, according to a 1998 study conducted at the School of Medicine, West Virginia University, Morgantown, West Virginia. The increases were detected in blood tests done forty-eight hours after an exercise session.

This study was consistent with previous studies on men, which reported increases in HDL after moderate exercise bouts lasting less than two hours. But the subfractions of HDL that may cause the rise of HDL may be different in women than in men, the researchers said. (See *British Journal of Sports Medicine,* March 1998, pp. 63–67.)

The message in this study seems clear: All women who have any concern whatsoever about their cholesterol should engage in moderate endurance exercise. You can improve your risk profile only if you lower your total or LDL cholesterol or raise your levels of HDL.

Problem: High risk of premature death from cardiovascular disease among sedentary, postmenopausal women.

Solution for Women: Moderate exercise.

Women who exercise after menopause also enjoy extra health benefits, including protection from premature death from cardiovascular disease and other causes of death, according to a 1997 report in the *Journal of the American Medical Association.* (See *JAMA,* vol. 277, April 23–30, 1997, pp. 1287–92.)

In this study, investigators from the University of Minnesota School of Public Health found that women who participated in moderate exercise, such as gardening or taking a long walk four or more times per week, were one-third less likely to die during the study than women who were sedentary. The study, which involved more than 40,000 women, aged 55 to 69, was conducted over a seven-year period, from 1986 through 1992.

In fact, the researchers discovered that the benefits could begin with just one walk. Women who took only one long walk per week—or the equivalent amount of other exercise—were 12 percent less likely to die than the sedentary women.

Problem: Low "good" HDL cholesterol in women smokers who are entering menopause, or who have gone through menopause.

Solution for Women: Stop smoking.

Smoking often depresses levels of "good" HDL cholesterol, a tendency that may be exacerbated for women, who lose their protective estrogen as they enter menopause and then move beyond it.

On the other hand, women who *quit* smoking at the menopausal stage of life may actually experience higher HDL cholesterol levels than do smokers or even nonsmokers, according to a 1998 study from the Department of Epidemiology, University of Pittsburgh. (See *American Journal of Public Health,* Jan. 1998, pp. 93–96.)

It's true that women who stop smoking during menopause or just afterward may gain weight. But the lower cardiovascular risk that comes with eliminating cigarettes offsets any increased risk associated with carrying the extra pounds.

Some Qualifications on Estrogen

An informal rule I follow in my practice says, "No drug is perfect"—and estrogen is certainly no exception. Although there is evidence that hormone replacement therapy, which includes estrogen, can lower cardiovascular risk for some menopausal women, other women apparently don't enjoy this benefit.

An August 1998 study published in the *Journal of the American Medical Association* found that women with a history of heart disease who took an estrogen-progestin supplement (HRT, or hormone replacement therapy) suffered no fewer heart attacks over a four-year period than women who didn't take the supplement. In other words, the HRT therapy didn't work in reducing cardiovascular risk. (See *JAMA,* vol. 280, August 19, 1998, pp. 605–13.)

This finding contrasts with previous reports that women who take these estrogen supplements suffer up to

60 percent less heart disease than women who are not on the supplements.

This report has raised questions among many practicing physicians who have been aggressive about prescribing HRT. But some ways have been suggested to distinguish between these two sets of findings.

For example, a number of experts have emphasized that the 1998 *JAMA* study involved patients with preexisting heart disease. It may be that those with the cardiovascular problems were too far along in their disease for the estrogen to have had a significant effect.

Right now most scientists and physicians seem to feel that HRT is worthwhile to prevent cardiovascular disease in high-risk women who have no symptoms or personal history of vessel or heart disease. But clearly, further research is needed in this area.

In the meantime, my own recommendations can be stated this way:

In general, women *with* a personal history of heart disease who are not currently on HRT should probably avoid the estrogen-progestin regimen because of the recent study showing no cardiovascular benefits and possibly some dangers. Of course, any final decision on this issue should be made only after you have consulted with your physician, who understands the details of your medical history.

Those with multiple cardiovascular risk factors or a family history of heart disease—but *without* personal history of the disease—may want to make use of HRT. But first they should try to modify all possible risk factors. Here's a summary of ways to modify these factors:

- Lower your elevated cholesterol;

- Lower your high blood pressure, either through lifestyle changes or medications;

- Stop cigarette smoking;

- Engage in regular, moderate exercise; and

- Control any tendency you may have toward diabetes.

If a woman without heart disease is unable or unwilling to change these risk factors, then HRT may be in order.

Finally, before we leave these topics that are "especially for women," I want to summarize some special distinctions—including telltale signs and symptoms—that may set women apart when heart disease strikes.

Is There a Gender Difference in Heart Disease?

Although there is wide variation in how heart attacks may occur, differences do sometimes appear along gender-related lines. One important distinction I've observed during my decades of medical practice is that a woman's heart disease symptoms *may be less intense* than a man's. Also, a woman's heart attack *may be more likely to be mistaken for some other health problem.*

So women should always be especially alert to unusual feelings and sensations that are not quite typical. Here are some examples:

- Relatively mild but continuing or recurring pains in the middle part of the chest (i.e., mild angina pains, which result from a reduced flow of blood and oxygen to the heart). You may erroneously believe these pains are the result of indigestion.

- Somewhat sharper pains, tightness, or numbness in the middle of the chest.

• Numbness or tightness that reaches up into the jaw or down through the left arm.

• Frequent breathlessness, which may become so intense during sleep that you wake up in the middle of the night, gasping for air.

• Dizziness or lightheadedness.

• Fainting episodes.

• Frequent fatigue, which may make it impossible for you to pursue your daily schedule.

• Recurring nausea or other gastrointestinal disturbances.

• Rapid heartbeats.

• Swelling of the ankles or lower legs.

(Sources for this information include the American Heart Association; Dr. Elizabeth Ross, coauthor of *Healing the Female Heart;* and the online Heart Information Network at *www.heartinfo.org.*)

Obviously, any of these signs and symptoms may have nothing to do with a heart attack. Your feelings of indigestion may *really be* indigestion! Or a sense of numbness or tightness in the left arm may be the result of fatigue or stress.

I recall one young patient, in her mid-thirties, who became frightened that she might be having heart problems when numbness and tightness in her left arm made it difficult for her to use her computer keyboard. Yet a series of tests—and some intense interviewing about her lifestyle and work habits—revealed that she had just been working too hard and had been under too much deadline pressure during a particularly stressful three-week period at her job.

Still, I respect such concerns. If you have any questions about whether you're confronting cardiovascular problems, I would recommend that you check with your doctor. A much-needed medical exam is preferable to neglecting a possibly serious condition—and suffering the consequences.

When a heart attack hits, men typically—but certainly not always—tend to have more pronounced symptoms than women. These may include intense crushing or squeezing pain in the middle of the chest (at the sternum), which may continue for several minutes, then recede and then return again. Or there may be an unusual sense of "fullness" in the chest, or nagging pain or numbness in the shoulders, neck, or arms (especially the left arm).

On the other hand, men, like women, may become faint, lightheaded, or dizzy. Or they may experience heavy or unusual sweating, shortness of breath, nausea, or an unusually fast heartbeat.

In any event, even though there frequently are gender differences, I don't want to overemphasize them. The symptoms for a particular man may be exactly the same as for a particular woman. Or symptoms may not be present at all. For example, both men and women may have silent heart attacks, which give no warning, even though they may be preparing the way for a later attack that ends in sudden death.

The fitness and running guru Jim Fixx—who was a friend of mine, though not a patient—had several silent heart attacks before he died in 1984 at age 52 of a massive coronary event during a training run in Vermont. I know he had those prior heart attacks because scar tissue on his heart, which was uncovered during his autopsy, confirmed the fact.

In other situations, the symptoms may be so mild—such as feelings of fatigue accompanied by a slight tightness or sense of discomfort in the chest—that the coronary event passes unrecognized for what it really is.

Many times the only way a patient or physician can learn whether a prior heart attack has occurred is for the patient to undergo a baseline exercise stress test and then to compare that initial electrocardiogram with later ones. Changes in the patterns of electrical activity in the heart will tend to show up during this kind of exam and may signal a serious blockage of blood flow to the heart, with death of some of the heart tissue. With this information in hand, the physician is in a stronger position to prescribe appropriate treatment.

In the last analysis, of course, your primary goal shouldn't be to recognize a heart attack when it occurs. Rather, you should concentrate right now on taking preventive measures to ensure that it never happens.

10

The Next Step in Cholesterol Control

As functional foods proliferate, it has become increasingly clear that they will soon make up a substantial proportion of our daily menus. There are even estimates that within the next few years, these products may constitute one-third or more of the foods we eat.

Many items, such as flour and cereals, are already fortified with folic acid, which reduces the risk of problem pregnancies, birth defects, and cardiovascular disease. Calcium has been added to orange juice and other products. Some popular cereals are packed full of megadoses of vitamins. Now, in even more dramatic fashion, cholesterol-lowering functional foods are quickly becoming a staple of many food plans.

With such innovations, we now stand at the beginning of an entirely new epoch in the prevention and treatment of disease. Furthermore, the powerful new products make it incumbent on each patient to work more closely than ever before with his or her physician.

No longer can any doctor or patient take it for granted that the only forum for promoting good health is the clinic or examining room. Instead, we have to assume that, in some cases, the dinner table may have just as great an impact on health. As a result, practicing physicians must become aware of exactly what their patients are eating and adjust their medications and medical procedures accordingly.

What does all this mean for the treatment of your cholesterol? The rise of functional foods has triggered an array of new questions—and "next steps"—in three key areas related to cholesterol control: treatment, diagnosis, and application of fast-breaking research.

The Next Step in Treatment

Our increasing ability to lower cholesterol so dramatically presents us with a surprising paradox: The prospect for the virtually unlimited ability to control blood lipids may give rise to an entirely different set of health concerns. To resolve this paradox, it's helpful to ask:

"How Low Should I Go with My Total and 'Bad' LDL Cholesterol?"

In general, the lower the levels you can achieve with your total and LDL cholesterol, the better—but there may be limits. With the exponential power of functional foods *and* medications now at our disposal, some have worried that perhaps we are in danger of toying with nature too much. They wonder if we may inadvertently reduce cholesterol below a healthy level and in effect cause the treatments to backfire on our health.

Here are a few of the concerns that have emerged from various observations and studies:

● **Low cholesterol levels have been linked to violent behavior.** In a 1998 review article published in the *Annals of Internal Medicine* and summarized in *Internal Medicine Alert* (April 29, 1998, p. 64), scientists who studied 167 journal articles concluded that there is indeed a consistent relationship between very low cholesterol levels and violence.

The reason? Experts have speculated that very low cholesterol levels may result in a reduced amount of the neurotransmitter serotonin in the central nervous system. Serotonin is associated with remaining calm and in control of oneself during the stresses and strains of daily life. At this point, however, there are no studies that have actually established a *causal* link between low cholesterol and violence.

● **Cholesterol-lowering drugs may dull your mental edge.** A study presented on November 10, 1997, at a meeting in Orlando of the American Heart Association, reported that certain of the statin drugs (described in Chapter 7) seem to reduce slightly the physical dexterity and attention spans of patients.

The University of Pittsburgh scientists who conducted the study tested participants by having them perform simple tests, such as putting small pegs into slots on a board. Those on the medication finished two seconds slower on average than those who were not medicated. (See *New York Times,* Nov. 11, 1997, p. B13.)

Other studies have indicated that those with very low cholesterol levels are more likely to die violently as a result of auto accidents and suicides. The scientists speculate that too-low cholesterol levels might reduce levels of vitamin A and other nutrients, which the brain needs to produce necessary proteins that "signal" the presence of danger.

But they caution that for most people, the dip in cholesterol levels is so little that no one should consider dropping his or her medications just to gain a barely perceptible mental edge. The danger from high cholesterol is far greater than from the uncertain impact of very low cholesterol or drug therapy.

• **Excessively low cholesterol levels are associated with higher death rates from cancer and other lethal diseases.** One reason for this may *not* be that diseases, such as cancer, are caused by low cholesterol. Rather, low cholesterol may just be a by-product of the disease. In other words, the chronic disease causes the low cholesterol—not the other way around. (See *New England Journal of Medicine,* July 8, 1993, author's reply letter, p. 138.)

So how are we to answer the question, "How low should you go with your cholesterol?"

First of all, I would certainly argue that preventing cardiovascular disease must be given a priority over any worry that somehow a health problem might develop from very low cholesterol. In other words, no one on cholesterol-lowering therapy should shy away from eating functional foods, going on a low-fat diet, or taking a prescribed medication simply because of the remote possibility that these measures might cause a minor drop in mental acuity.

An important related issue—and perhaps the most important question—is how low do you have to go with your LDL to continue to derive the maximum benefit of risk reduction for cardiovascular disease?

One study from the Harvard Medical School showed that risks declined until "bad" LDL cholesterol reached a measurement of 124 but didn't decline at levels below that. Another report from Aker Hospital in Oslo, Norway, found benefits when LDL levels dropped below 100. (See *Lancet,* April 25, 1998, p. 1257; *Circulation,* vol. 97, 1998, pp. 1436–60.)

As a result of such studies, the National Cholesterol Education Program, which is endorsed by the American Heart Association, recommends that individuals reduce their "bad" LDL cholesterol levels at least down to 130. Those with heart disease should make LDL of 100 their goal.

Summing up these conclusions, Dr. Scott Grundy, Director of the Center for Human Nutrition at the University of Texas Southwestern Medical Center in Dallas, says that most heart disease patients with LDL above 130 should receive cholesterol-lowering drugs.

I agree with these recommendations. But I would also add that at this point there seems to be no reason for those without coronary or vessel disease to take their total cholesterol much below 180, or "bad" LDL cholesterol much below 120. On the other hand, those with cardiovascular disease *should* have LDL cholesterol below 100 and total cholesterol below 160.

But of course, most people still worry most about getting their cholesterol levels down to normal—and one of those groups that has come under increasing scrutiny in recent years is the elderly.

Should Those in Their Late Sixties or Older—Who Have Never Had Symptoms of Heart Disease—Worry About Treating Cholesterol?

A controversy has developed during the 1990s about whether older people—those from about age 65 on up—should be treated for elevated cholesterol levels. Here's the way the discussion has gone:

Researchers from the Honolulu Heart Program concluded in a 1990 study that total cholesterol is an independent predictor of coronary heart disease among men older than age 65. As a result, they said, elevated cholesterol should be treated in elderly men, just as it is in middle-aged men. (See *Journal of the American Medical Association,* Jan. 19, 1990, pp. 393–96.)

The researchers in this investigation followed 1,480 men, who were 65 or older, for 12 years. The incidence of cardiovascular disease increased significantly as the average total cholesterol levels moved from 190 mg/dl up to 240 and higher.

Although earlier findings by the renowned Framingham study showed that there was no link between elevated cholesterol and heart disease in elderly men, the Honolulu researchers distinguished their findings in several ways.

For one thing, the Honolulu scientists followed their subjects for a longer period of time, so they were able to identify disease that developed later. Also, the Honolulu researchers speculated that the Framingham study participants may have received more rigorous treatment of their disease than those in the Hawaiian investigation. Among other things, physicians saw the Framingham participants more often.

But the issue wasn't laid to rest with this report.

A 1994 investigation by scientists from the Yale University School of Medicine studied the cholesterol–heart disease connection in 997 men and women, who averaged 79 years of age. They concluded that their findings with this group did *not* support the idea that either high total cholesterol or low "good" HDL cholesterol was an important risk factor for cardiovascular disease, death by heart attack, or death from other causes. (See *Journal of the American Medical Association,* Nov. 2, 1994, pp. 1335–40.)

An editorial in *JAMA*, published in the same issue as this study, made these recommendations:

First, "younger elderly people"—men and women up to their mid-seventies—may be treated for elevated cholesterol if they already have signs of hardening of the arteries, or atherosclerosis. Also, it's appropriate to treat men in this age category who have risk factors that put them at a high risk for death from cardiovascular disease.

But the editorial writers did not support the treatment of most elderly women in this "young elderly" category for elevated cholesterol. Furthermore, they said that elderly patients, those in their late seventies and older, should as a general rule not be screened or treated for high blood cholesterol at all.

But even this strong position by *JAMA* didn't end the debate.

A 1995 report from the National Institute on Aging concluded that low "good" HDL cholesterol can predict coronary-heart-disease death in people who are older than 70. On the other hand, this report did not find a link between high total cholesterol and fatal heart disease in older men. But the researchers did suggest that high cholesterol might be a risk factor for older women. (*JAMA*, August 16, 1995, pp. 539–44.)

This back-and-forth discussion among the medical researchers often confuses the average elderly person who is trying to figure out what to do. To clear up the confusion, here's what I think is the best recommendation:

There is considerable evidence that high cholesterol is a significant risk factor for fatal cardiovascular disease in a number of groups who are over 65 years of age. So I recommend that high or unbalanced cholesterol should be treated for those up to age 80 in the same way that it's treated for younger people.

Also, if you've been undergoing treatment before age

80, you should probably continue with the same medications, functional foods, or low-fat diet that you've been following.

On the other hand, if you're already past 80 and you've never been diagnosed with or treated for cardiovascular problems, don't worry now! The chances are, if you haven't had any problems up to this point, you won't confront any at all.

At the other end of the age spectrum, increasing attention is being paid to the young—with an important issue that can be posed this way:

Should Cholesterol Testing and Treatment Begin with Children?

The answer to this question is a qualified yes, according to an insightful editorial in the June 4, 1998, issue of the *New England Journal of Medicine* (vol. 338, no. 23, pp. 1690–91).

The author notes that early in the next century, cardiovascular disease will most likely be the number-one killer throughout the world. As a result, it's important to step up our preventive health efforts for children and young adults—and that includes a significant increase in efforts to educate parents and children about the mechanisms and dangers of cholesterol.

For example, many young people—or adults, for that matter—don't focus on the fact that the epidemic of cigarette smoking among adolescents is associated with high cholesterol levels. Yet this habit is a key factor in raising the risk for early cardiovascular disease and heart attacks.

The editorial also suggests that more attention be paid to educating children and their parents about the importance of managing other cardiovascular risk factors, such going on a low-fat diet, engaging in regular physical activity, and eliminating obesity.

On the other hand, the author is wary of mass screening of children for cholesterol levels because of the cost and likely inefficiencies of such testing. But he cites approvingly recommendations of the National Cholesterol Education Program that children in high-risk families— that is, those with a family history of hypercholesterolemia, or genetically high cholesterol—be tested. Also, he believes that young adults should undergo testing for cholesterol and blood pressure levels.

My own variation on these recommendations can be stated this way:

- Mass, governmentally financed cholesterol screening for all children does seem to be going too far. But all children who have a family history of high cholesterol or a family history of heart disease before 50 years of age should be checked by age five or six—perhaps as part of a national school clinic program.

- Also, on a private basis, parents should consider having their child's pediatrician do a blood test on their child at an early age—say, by age five or six—to establish a baseline cholesterol reading. This way if a problem shows up, you will be in a position to do something about it before the buildup of vessel plaque becomes serious. If there is no problem, the next test can be done when the child becomes a teenager.

- All young adults, beginning at about age 18, should undergo a cholesterol blood test.

- All parents should be educated and encouraged to take steps to lower their children's risk of cardiovascular disease. This means promoting a low-fat diet, regular exercise, and a healthy, nonobese level of body fat.

Another area of concern about high cholesterol has been its link to other diseases—such as diabetes and insulin resistance. The question about the insulin connection can be posed this way:

What Is the Connection Between High Blood Fats and a Tendency Toward High Blood Sugar or Diabetes?

The answer to this complex question—which is currently being explored in a variety of scientific studies—begins with knowing your blood glucose (sugar) level, which should be one of the items on your regular blood test. The desired glucose range is generally 80 to 120 mg/dl.

Anything above that could indicate *insulin resistance* and a tendency toward diabetes. Also, either an abnormal glucose result or a personal history of diabetes also puts you at greater risk for heart disease.

> **Note:** *Insulin resistance* refers to a reduced effectiveness of the body's insulin in lowering sugar levels in the blood.

What's the connection with blood fats? Recent research has established a possible link between insulin resistance and elevated blood lipids, such as cholesterol and triglycerides, which are associated with cardiovascular disease. Furthermore, even though insulin problems are commonly associated with diabetics, some studies have indicated that even nondiabetic people with insulin resistance are also at higher risk for cardiovascular disease.

Dr. Scott Grundy cites the 1991 Paris Prospective Study to suggest this link. He notes that some forms of coronary heart disease may arise from a grouping or "constellation" of metabolic abnormalities—including elevated triglycerides, insulin resistance, and obesity.

Also, a line of research findings has suggested that higher levels of certain blood-related cardiovascular risk factors—including high total cholesterol, high "bad" LDL cholesterol, and high triglycerides—may be the first signs of the onset of diabetes in prediabetic individuals. (See *Lipid Management,* vol. 1, no. 2, Fall 1996, pp. 7–8.)

This insulin connection—which is becoming an important predictor for blood-fat abnormalities and cardiovascular risk—brings us to another "next step" area of cholesterol control: the exciting new developments in diagnostic techniques.

The Next Step in Diagnosis

A few important developments are currently being implemented or are on the immediate horizon in the diagnosis of cholesterol-related heart and vessel problems.

The first concerns innovations applied to the traditional stress test—which may turn it into a "super stress test." The second involves the fast growth of dramatic computer-imaging technology, which permits you and your physician to look directly into your blood vessels to identify blockages.

Toward a "Super Stress Test"?

Some fascinating developments that have just emerged in the medical literature indicate that the traditional stress test—which helps identify vessel blockages—can be transformed into a "super stress test" with even broader diagnostic power.

To understand the "super" variation, you first must grasp the basics of the traditional test:

A traditional stress test, which provides an *exercise electrocardiogram,* is essential before you embark on a new exercise program. In fact, I routinely order the traditional test as part of every annual medical exam for men over 40 years of age and women over 50 because, when performed by qualified medical personnel, it can be quite accurate in predicting blockages to blood vessels. (These are caused by oxidized cholesterol that sticks to vessel walls as plaque.)

This part of your exam involves having at least ten electrodes affixed to your chest. These are rubber pads attached to small pieces of metal, which in turn are connected to an electrocardiograph. This device produces an electrocardiogram, or a tracing on a roll of paper that records the electrical activity of your heartbeats.

Then you step on a treadmill or climb onto a stationary bicycle. During the test, you'll begin at a comfortably slow pace, and gradually the level of difficulty will increase. You should exercise to exhaustion—or until you approach your maximum heart rate and can't sustain the pace any longer.

Why is the test so important?

Many times, physicians can't see any problems with your heart until high demands—or physical stresses—are placed upon it. At the more intense levels of activity, skipped and irregular heartbeats may signal underlying clogging or disease of the blood vessels.

At the Cooper Institute, we have recently completed analysis of a study involving 25,662 men, followed for over eight years. This investigation showed clearly that a classic abnormal stress test—with *ischemic ST changes* reflected on the electrocardiogram—was a better predictor of a future fatal heart attack than any of the standard coronary risk factors. These other risk factors included high cholesterol, elevated blood pressure, cigarette smoking, and a family history of heart disease.

Our investigation revealed that a man with an abnormal stress electrocardiogram and no coronary risk factors was twice as likely to die of a heart attack than was a man with three or more coronary risk factors and a normal stress electrocardiogram!

In other words, an abnormal stress electrocardiogram may be the most important of all the risk factors, even though most physicians are saying you don't need a stress test unless you have one or more risk factors. (This summary is based on unpublished data from the Aerobics Center Longitudinal Study, Cooper Institute for Aerobics Research.)

But now we appear to be on the verge of new breakthroughs that will make the traditional stress test an even more effective tool in uncovering cardiovascular disease.

The key development is the Cambridge Heart Inc.'s Alternans test, recently approved by the Food and Drug Administration. Studies in *Circulation, The New England Journal of Medicine,* and other leading journals have revealed that *T-wave alternans,* or electrical fluctuations from heartbeat to heartbeat on an electrocardiogram, can be a good predictor of *ventricular fibrillation,* or an irregular heartbeat that may result in sudden death. (See *New England Journal of Medicine,* vol. 330, Jan. 27, 1994, pp. 235–41; *Circulation,* March 16, 1999, pp. 1385–94.)

Scientists have discovered that an effective means to identify these T-wave alternans is to employ a special kind of stress test, with high-performance electrodes that reduce noise and increase sensitivity of heartbeat measurements. (See *Journal of Electrocardiology,* vol. 29 suppl., 1996, pp. 46–51.)

Once offending electrical fluctuations in the heart have been identified, the patient can receive an implanted *defibrillator,* which prevents the heartbeats from becoming irregular. With this device, there is a much lower risk that those with ventricular fibrillation will suffer a sudden lethal heart attack.

In the past, to identify the T-wave alternans, it has been

necessary to employ *electrophysiologic testing,* a highly invasive, relatively risky, and expensive technique involving the surgical implantation of electrodes in the heart. But now, with the new super stress test, the projected cost for the procedure is about $350, or approximately $100 more than a regular stress test.

I'm quite encouraged by this advance in stress-test technology because I myself have picked up many cases of heart and vessel disease from the *regular* stress test alone. Also, I've found that the degree of accuracy in predicting disease rises considerably when the stress test is combined with tests done using the Ultrafast CT scan—another new diagnostic technique.

Cholesterol and the Computer-Imaging Frontier

In the past, the only way that we could really peer into the blood vessels was to conduct the invasive coronary arteriogram. This procedure involves injecting a dye into the heart through the blood vessels and then taking pictures of the heart and coronary vessels to see if there are *occlusions,* or a narrowing of vessels as a result of buildup of plaque.

Though still considered in many quarters as the "gold standard" test to determine vessel blockage, this technique is typically used only for the highest-risk patients. For one thing, it costs a great deal. Also, there is some degree of risk, in that the catheter that is inserted in the vessels may inadvertently break off pieces of plaque and promote blockages.

Now, however, a new noninvasive technique has become available in a few diagnostic facilities around the country, including the Cooper Clinic. This is Imatron's Ultrafast CT scan—a machine that uses *electron beam computed tomography* (EBCT). The scan is able to identify "hard" calcification in the arteries and has also been useful in helping us pick up tumors involving internal organs, such as the liver and kidneys.

The basic technique is to hook up two electrodes to the patient's chest without requiring the person to disrobe. Then the individual lies down in an open tubelike device—which, I might add, is *so* open that it hasn't caused problems for anyone I know with claustrophobia.

The scan takes about eight to ten minutes to complete and employs low-grade radiation, which is about the radiation required for a standard abdominal X-ray. Computer-generated pictures are immediately available for physician and patient to review. Perhaps most important of all, the patient can learn the extent of calcification of his vessels and his likely risk for a heart attack. These results are reported as a coronary-artery-calcification number.

There have also been recent reports that regular CT (computed tomography) scanners, which are used in most hospitals, can be combined with an electrocardiograph machine to produce images that are similar to those of the more expensive Ultrafast scanner. If this new testing technique proves as effective as the Ultrafast CT, diagnosis through computer imaging could become much more widely available.

How well does this new technology work? Let me illustrate.

One patient in his fifties, whom I'll call Chuck, came into my office complaining about feelings of "suffocation" he had experienced walking while on vacation at a 9,000-foot elevation in the mountains. He also said he had gone off his walking exercise program because of a joint problem and was experiencing a blurring of vision in one of his eyes.

A visit to an optometrist revealed no eye problem, and I suspected that the underlying cause might be a blockage in his blood vessels. I ordered a stress test—which came back with a terrible EKG (electrocardiogram). But I wanted to be sure before I scheduled him for more invasive tests, such as a coronary arteriogram.

Chuck learned from the Ultrafast CT scan that he had experienced a 40 percent increase in his calcification score during the past year. Clearly, we had to take immediate action. He had a coronary arteriogram that showed severe disease necessitating a multiple bypass procedure, and even though he had some trouble during recovery, he was finally discharged. Now, several months later, he is still showing none of the symptoms he was experiencing before.

As a result of success in diagnosing patients like Chuck, I've been making increasing use of a combination of stress testing plus Imatron's Ultrafast CT scanner. I find that if I combine both tests—especially with those patients who have an equivocal or uncertain stress test—I can improve my testing specificity and sensitivity. By using the Ultrafast CT, I have achieved a greater degree of accuracy in predicting cardiovascular problems than was possible in the past.

To sum up the advantages, I've found that the new device is:

- A superior predictor of current or future artery disease.

- A good way to determine whether or not a patient with high cholesterol should be treated aggressively with medications.

- A way to tell if *reversal* of calcification of the arteries is occurring—which is a real possibility if the patient has LDL cholesterol below 120, according to scientific studies.

- A possible noninvasive replacement for diagnosis done with invasive and riskier coronary arteriography.

• A highly useful, accurate, and *speedy* means of checking on whether certain symptoms, such as chest pains, indicate the occurrence of a heart attack, according to Mayo Clinic studies that have been done with emergency room patients.

Even though these diagnostic innovations are already available in some clinics and hospitals, they are also part of the incredible research explosion in this field.

The Next Step in Research

As we have already seen, some of the most exciting cholesterol research in recent years has focused on functional foods—and there is no doubt that this movement will continue apace. But important research is also focusing on the nature of some of the intriguing subcomponents of cholesterol, and efforts are being made to translate this "pure" research into practical treatments and medications.

The "Tough Little Bad Guys" in LDL Cholesterol

Apparently some forms of "bad" LDL cholesterol are worse than others. A number of scientific papers in the last couple of years have focused on special dangers posed by the small size and high density of certain particles of LDL cholesterol—or what I sometimes call the "tough little bad guys in your blood."

For example, a report in the June 24, 1998, issue of *JAMA* noted that there is a higher prevalence of small, dense LDL molecules in patients who have ischemic heart disease. This condition, which results from narrowed coronary arteries that feed blood and oxygen to the heart, is often the forerunner of heart attacks (vol. 297, no. 24, pp. 1955–61).

Also, these researchers reasoned that the small, dense LDL particles might cause clogging of the arteries for a couple of reasons. First, they may be most susceptible to becoming oxidized through the action of free radicals (unstable oxygen molecules). This process causes the LDL to stick to vessel walls and contribute to the buildup of plaque.

Second, the little LDL molecules may be less likely to hook up with LDL receptors on the vessel walls—a tendency that keeps them from making healthy contributions to the body's cell development and other productive functions.

Is there any way to test for these small LDL particles?

In a recent article in *Physician and Sportsmedicine* (Vol. 26, no. 11, November 1998, pp. 62–63), two of my colleagues at the Cooper Wellness Program and the Cooper Clinic—Dr. Tedd L. Mitchell and Dr. Larry W. Gibbons—recommended additional cholesterol tests for some people.

In particular, they suggested that for patients with coronary artery disease that continues to worsen despite decreases in "bad" LDL cholesterol, the levels of the small, dense LDL particles should be measured. These molecules are called *small dense LDL cholesterol,* or SDLDL-C for short.

Even though these tests are expensive, the authors say they may be worth the cost for patients with these characteristics:

- A pronounced family history of early coronary artery disease, even without other risk factors.

- Levels of "bad" LDL cholesterol that are normal or close to normal.

- An increase of plaque buildup in the arteries even if LDL levels are normal and other cardiovascular risk factors are under control.

The authors point out that the small LDL molecules may not respond well to statin drugs, but they may be controlled with niacin and a well-planned low-cholesterol, low-fat diet.

The Ongoing "ApoB" Drama

Another possible risk related to cholesterol involves *Apolipoprotein B,* or ApoB—which has continued to be an important player in the cholesterol drama, even since I described this particle in some detail in *Controlling Cholesterol.*

In brief, ApoB, the protein portion of the LDL molecule, may be the most accurate estimate or marker for LDL that's circulating in the bloodstream. Also, some experts believe there may be a causal link between the amount of ApoB that is circulating in a person's blood and the likelihood that the person will develop atherosclerosis, or clogging of the arteries.

So in the future, when technology is more generally available to test for ApoB in a routine blood test, we may turn to this measurement as one of our best predictors of heart disease. Instead of just knowing your levels of total cholesterol, "bad" LDL cholesterol, and "good" HDL cholesterol, you'll also have to be aware of your ApoB.

At the same time that we fine-tune our diagnosis procedures, we can expect researchers to continue to try to develop new ways to target ApoB, as well as the little, dense LDL particles, for special treatment. At this point, our primary treatment options involve the new functional foods, a low-fat diet, and if necessary, drugs such as the statins.

The "Ugly Cholesterol" Controversy

A somewhat more controversial topic concerns a subcomponent of cholesterol known in technical terms as *lipoprotein(a),* or Lp(a) for short. More popularly, this particle has been dubbed "ugly cholesterol" because some studies have associated its presence in the blood with an exceptionally high risk of developing heart disease.

For example, the Framingham study researchers reported in 1996 on a study involving Lp(a), which they had conducted of 2,191 men, aged 20 to 54, during a 15-year follow-up period. (See *JAMA,* vol. 276, no. 7, August 21, 1996, pp. 544–48.) They concluded that elevated levels of Lp(a) are an independent risk factor for the development of premature coronary heart disease in men. Furthermore, they identified this blood particle as comparable in danger to a total cholesterol level of 240 mg/dl or higher, or a "good" HDL level of less than 35.

But not all scientists agree with this conclusion.

A forceful contrary argument appeared in another *JAMA* study published earlier, on November 10, 1993 (pp. 2195–99). In that report, researchers from Harvard evaluated nearly 15,000 male doctors who participated in the Physicians' Health Study. They found no evidence of any association between Lp(a) levels and the risk of future heart attacks. Furthermore, they declared that their data did not support the use of Lp(a) levels as a screening tool to determine cardiovascular risk.

What can we conclude about this dispute?

At this point, there is agreement that even if Lp(a) turns out to be an independent risk factor for cardiovascular disease, we don't have the means at hand to test effectively for it. More importantly, we have no way to treat the problem.

The best advice I can give is just to keep an eye on developments with Lp(a), but don't worry about it right now for purposes of treatment—at least not until we have more solid information to act on. In any case, I fully expect that the current treatments we're using—including the growing array of functional foods—will take care of any problems we may finally trace to the operation of "ugly" cholesterol.

What Will Be the Successor to the Statin Drugs?

No one can answer this question for certain. But one promising new type of drug that may soon dominate the market comes from the field of genetics.

It has been estimated that within fifteen years, we may be able to lower cholesterol and prevent heart attacks by applying medications that interrupt the operation of certain genes that play a role in forming cholesterol. (See *Wall Street Journal,* Oct. 23, 1998, p. B1; also the Oct. 23, 1998, issue of *Science.*)

These new drugs that are now being studied interfere with the activity of a human protein known as MTP. In animal studies, when certain drugs block MTP, they also reduce the levels of cholesterol and other blood fats. MTP plays a role in producing lipids, such as cholesterol. Human tests in this area are already under way by Bristol-Myers, which was the first to pursue this research. Bayer, Glaxo, and Pfizer are also doing human studies, and Johnson & Johnson and a Japanese company are planning tests as well.

If these studies prove that the MTP-blocking medications are effective and safe and involve minimal or no side effects, we may soon have another powerful weapon in our cholesterol-management arsenal.

It's almost certain, however, that these new drugs will be able to be adjusted and reduced in dosage through the functional food strategy we've been discussing throughout this book. In other words, those with cholesterol problems will first try lifestyle changes and, next, functional foods like Benecol, before they turn to medications—including the new MTP blockers. Furthermore, it's likely that because the MTP cholesterol-lowering mechanism is different from that of the other drugs, the new medications may be combined with some of the older drugs to enhance the total effect.

Up to this point, we've covered a great deal of ground, as we have explored many avenues for controlling cholesterol the natural way. There's one more area of natural remedies to cover: vitamin and dietary supplements.

11

The Scoop on Supplements

I am often asked which vitamin and dietary supplements are effective in managing cholesterol, and which, if any of these natural remedies, I recommend to my patients. So in this chapter I share the scoop on the following supplements: vitamin E, vitamin C, cholestin, lecithin, garlic, fish oil, and flaxseed.

Vitamins

Yes, vitamin supplements can help improve your cholesterol picture, and yes, I consider them functional foods.

A solid link has been established in recent years between controlling cholesterol the natural way and a wise use of nutritional supplements—particularly those classed as antioxidants. The weight of scientific evidence now supports the existence of a strong association between the destructive work of free radicals (unstable oxygen molecules that create oxidative stress) on cholesterol and the buildup of plaque in the blood vessels. This clogging or hardening of the arteries—which we know as atherosclerosis or arteriosclerosis—is the primary cause of heart attacks and strokes.

In brief, here is a reminder about the step-by-step biological drama that may be occurring in your body.

First, free radicals in the blood and tissues—which may be generated from a variety of sources, including cigarette smoke, inflammation, disease, stress, and excessive exercise—attack free-floating "bad" LDL molecules that have failed to "latch on" to receptors in the cells. The most vulnerable LDL molecules may be small, dense ones, which I sometimes call the "tough little bad guys" in your blood. (See the description on pages 200–01.)

Current thinking suggests that after the free radicals "wound" an LDL molecule, the LDL is consumed by white blood cells, known as *macrophages.* The combination macrophage-LDL particle then swells up into a *foam cell,* which sticks in the artery wall.

As more of the foam cells pile up on one another, plaque develops in the artery, and the vessel begins to close down. Coronary arteries—or those that feed blood to the heart—may become so clogged up (or occluded) that the blood flow to the heart is shut off. This produces ischemia, or a lack of sufficient oxygen to the heart tissues—and a heart attack (myocardial infarction, or MI) is the end result.

What can you do to head off the vessel disease caused by attacks launched by free radicals on your LDL cholesterol?

Vitamin E

Research offers increasing support for the idea that an effective antidote to atherosclerosis is antioxidants—preferably natural vitamin E (listed in technical terms on the labels of vitamin bottles as "d-alpha-tocopherol").

Note: *Natural* vitamin E has only the letter "d" on the label, whereas synthetic vitamin E has a "dl" designation. What you want is the "d" or natural type.

A 1997 editorial in *Circulation* confirmed that vitamins and antioxidants are effective in reducing the progression of coronary artery disease and nonfatal heart attacks. The authors noted that two studies indicated that prolonged vitamin E intake was able to reduce the risk of coronary disease. (See *Circulation,* vol. 96, 1997, pp. 3264–65.)

A 1998 study—conducted by Dr. Ishwarlal Jialal and colleagues from the Center for Human Nutrition, University of Texas Southwestern Medical Center, Dallas—focused on how different amounts of vitamin E worked in preventing the oxidation of "bad" LDL cholesterol. (See *American Journal of Cardiology,* vol. 81, Jan. 15, 1998, pp. 231–33.) These researchers found that taking 1200 IU per day of natural vitamin E is more potent in decreasing the susceptibility of "bad" LDL cholesterol to oxidation than taking 400 IU per day. Also, different groups of investigators have discovered that it takes about eight weeks for vitamin E to have a significant effect on the LDL oxidative process.

This study, when taken with others that have been done on vitamin E and cardiovascular disease, prompts me to give these recommendations:

The average adult, up to age 50, should be taking at least 400 IU of natural vitamin E (d-alpha tocopherol) every day. As much as 1,200 per day may be appropriate if you are a heavy exerciser or are exposed to the attacks of unusual levels of free radicals, such as through cigarette smoke or high stress.

And Add Vitamin C

In addition to vitamin E, there is evidence that vitamin C may work synergistically to increase the power of E, or may even have a beneficial effect on its own in lowering cholesterol in some people. With these and other possible benefits that aren't even related to cholesterol, I recommend that my average adult patient take in at least 1,000 mg per day in the form of supplements. Significant amounts can also be obtained through a number of foods, such as raw papaya, raw sweet yellow pepper, fresh orange juice, broccoli, and cantaloupe.

The full impact of taking relatively large doses of antioxidant vitamins on heart disease is still being explored. But there is undoubtedly much more that we'll learn about the vitamin story as new research comes to light.

For example, a number of years ago, a couple of isolated but intriguing studies associated vitamin C levels in the blood with lower cholesterol levels. The effect was especially pronounced in people who either had high levels of blood cholesterol or had a low consumption of the vitamin in their diets.

More recently, a 1998 study in *Epidemiology* (vol. 9, pp. 316–21) reported that a 0.5 percent increase in vitamin C in the blood was associated with an 11 percent reduction in cardiovascular disease, including heart problems and stroke. A related study revealed that those with the highest consumption of vitamin C had a 25-to-50 percent reduction in cardiovascular deaths. (See *Clinical Pearls News,* August 1998, p. 125.)

As such findings continue to emerge in the scientific literature, I become increasingly convinced about the validity of my vitamin recommendations. These antioxidants may be more important than we realize in actually lowering cholesterol levels—not to mention preventing oxidation of "bad" LDL molecules.

Dietary Supplements

Cholestin

In general, I don't recommend that you take Cholestin—a red yeast rice also known as hongqu, hong qu, or hung-chu—to lower your cholesterol.

At one point, the FDA moved to block the sale of Cholestin, which contains the same active ingredient as lovastatin (marketed as the drug Mevacor). The makers of Cholestin prevailed over the FDA in court, but I still have questions about how or whether the product should be used by the general consumer without medical supervision.

The product claims include the lowering of total cholesterol and the raising of "good" HDL cholesterol—and there is evidence that these benefits may indeed occur. Unfortunately, the FDA hasn't monitored the purity of Cholestin because it's sold as an herb or supplement. In fact, the FDA took the position that this substance is actually an unapproved drug, and that means government regulations can be applied.

In any event, products like Cholestin, if they are taken at all, should be used only under the recommendation and supervision of a qualified physician. Remember: This product apparently contains chemical properties similar to those of lovastatin—and also behaves like lovastatin. If something looks and acts like a drug, it probably is a drug and should be approached with the same caution.

Lecithin

I also don't think that taking a lecithin supplement will help improve cholesterol levels.

Some findings in animal studies suggest that supplements of lecithin—which are chemical compounds in the body consisting of phosphorus and fatty substances—

may be able to lower cholesterol levels. Specifically, a 1998 study of soy lecithin, which was fed to monkeys on a low-fat diet, showed that the lecithin could lower levels of total cholesterol significantly below levels achieved by a low-fat diet alone. (See *Atherosclerosis,* vol. 140, no. 1, Sept. 1998, pp. 147–53.) In the same study, hamsters on a soy lecithin regimen had lower total cholesterol and less pronounced fatty streaks on the aortic artery leading to the heart than hamsters not on the supplement.

But human studies haven't been so promising. In a June 1998 report in the *European Journal of Clinical Nutrition,* researchers from the Department of Nutrition, Potchefstroom University for Christian Higher Education, South Africa, concluded that lecithin treatments had no independent effects on any blood lipids—including serum total cholesterol, triglycerides, "bad" LDL cholesterol, or "good" HDL cholesterol (vol. 52, no. 6, pp. 419–24).

Similarly, an earlier study in the *American Journal of Clinical Nutrition* concluded there was no evidence for a specific effect of lecithin on blood cholesterol. Positive changes that did occur among participants who took the lecithin were attributed for the most part to changes in the patients' intake of dietary fat during the studies (vol. 49, no. 2, Feb. 1989, pp. 266–68).

In light of the results of these human studies, I must conclude that there isn't sufficient evidence at this point to rely on lecithin as a vehicle to lower or balance your cholesterol. Instead, stick to the tried-and-true dietary approaches discussed in chapter 3 and the recently proven nutriceutical possibilities outlined in chapters 4 to 8.

Garlic

Garlic is yet another natural remedy that presents us with a mixed picture when it comes to helping manage cholesterol levels. Some findings suggest that eating a clove of garlic each day will reduce levels of "bad" LDL cholesterol by as much as 9 percent, and one study has found that total cholesterol may drop by up to 20 percent. (See *Bottom Line Health,* vol. 12, no. 5, May 1998, p. 2; *Prostaglandins, Leukocytes and Essential Fatty Acids,* Sept. 1995, pp. 211–12.)

But a more recent 1998 study in the *Archives of Internal Medicine* (vol. 158, no. 11, pp. 1189–94) concluded that taking garlic powder tablets won't lower cholesterol in patients who have mildly elevated total cholesterol. In this study, the subjects had an average "bad" LDL level of 160 when they began the study, but blood tests at the end of the investigation revealed no significant changes.

The researchers did say, however, that further studies should be done to determine if there is something in garlic that may lower the risk of cardiovascular disease. One possibility they suggested is that garlic may reduce the tendency of blood platelets to adhere to one another and form life-threatening clots in the vessels.

Why the difference in the above studies?

It may be that the body responds differently to garlic powders as opposed to garlic cloves. Also, a reviewer in *Physician and Sportsmedicine* (vol. 26, no. 11, Nov. 1998, p. 24) suggested that previous studies of garlic and cholesterol have failed to consider the fact that the studies are usually done in conjunction with a low-fat diet. In other words, it may be the diet, not the garlic, that is lowering the cholesterol in the studies.

Fish Oil

Fish oil—especially the omega-3 fatty acids in deep sea fish, such as salmon, tuna, lake trout, mackerel, and herring—has been linked to a lower cardiovascular risk and lower rate of heart attack deaths.

A 1998 report in the *Journal of the American Medical Association* (vol. 279, pp. 23–28) focused on the fish consumption of more than 20,000 American doctors during an 11-year period. The researchers found that one fish meal a week was able to lower the risk of a sudden, fatal heart attack by 52 percent. One explanation offered was that the fatty acids in the fish decreased the risk of a fatal irregular beating of the heart. (See *Running & Fitness,* July 1998, p. 1.)

Another study, a 2-year investigation of male survivors of a heart attack, published in 1989 in *Lancet,* found that moderate consumption of fatty fish or fish oil decreased total deaths by 29 percent (vol. 2, p. 757). Also, there is evidence that omega-3 fatty acids in fish help lower triglycerides. (See *Bottom Line Health,* May 1998, p. 2.)

Finally, a fascinating 1998 study reported on men who took one of three supplements: fish oil alone, garlic powder alone, or fish oil plus garlic. The researchers found that the men on fish oil alone experienced no change in their cholesterol levels. Those who took the garlic alone had a 11.5 percent drop in their cholesterol—a finding, you'll note, that seems inconsistent with the study on garlic powder cited in the answer to the previous question. Those with the combination supplements—fish oil plus garlic powder—enjoyed a 12.2 percent drop in their total cholesterol. (See *Bottom Line Health,* vol. 12, no. 3, March 1998, p. 1.)

What's the message here? The benefits of garlic remain unclear. But there does seem to be some benefit in the omega-3 fatty acids that are found in fish. I always recommend that my patients stick to real fish, however, rather than the fish oil capsules.

Flaxseed

In several studies, flaxseed has been associated with a lowering of cholesterol—especially "bad" LDL cholesterol.

In a 3-week investigation conducted at the University of Toronto and reported in 1999 in the *American Journal of Clinical Nutrition* (vol. 69, March, pp. 395–402), 22 men and 7 postmenopausal women consumed muffins that contained either 50 grams per day of defatted flaxseed or wheat bran. The researchers found that those eating the flaxseed muffins experienced an average reduction in LDL cholesterol of 7.6 percent, and a reduction in total cholesterol of 4.6 percent.

In a 4-week study, also at the University of Toronto, young adults ate muffins containing 50 grams of flaxseed per day. Their LDL cholesterol dropped by up to 8 percent, and their weekly bowel movements increased by 30 percent. The researchers concluded that flaxseed could produce these benefits without compromising the subjects' antioxidant blood levels.

Studies done on rabbits have also shown benefits that may apply to humans. For example, an investigation at the University of Saskatchewan in Canada reported that a plant lignan, which is a component of flaxseed fiber, reduced atherosclerosis associated with high cholesterol in the animals. This effect was accompanied by a decrease in serum (blood) cholesterol, "bad" LDL cholesterol, and oxidation of lipids (fats) in the blood.

The best way to use flaxseed seems to be to consume the entire seed—which contains a considerable amount of soluble fiber. Both the fiber and omega-3 fatty acids, which are abundant in flaxseed, have been associated with a lower risk of coronary heart disease. (See *Environmental Nutrition,* December 1988, p. 7.)

Where can you get flaxseed? Most people buy it at

health food stores or order it through the mail. You can store whole flaxseed at room temperature for as long as a year, or you can refrigerate milled flaxseed in an airtight, opaque container for up to one month.

A dietary suggestion from the *Environmental Nutrition* article cited above is that you can grind up seeds with a coffee grinder and then add them to batter for pancakes and baked goods. You can mix whole seeds or ground seeds with cereal, yogurt—or even chew them. But you have to be sure to chew them well or you won't derive the full benefit.

Note: To take in an amount consistent with the best effects in the scientific studies cited above, you should try to eat the equivalent of about 50 grams of raw flaxseed per day.

I'm sure you still have questions you would like to put to me. That's why I'm giving you an opportunity to ask them in the following pages.

12

Answering Questions About Your Heart

Question: Can a designed functional food improve my health in any way other than by lowering or balancing my cholesterol?

Answer: Yes, there may indeed be other benefits, according to researchers W. H. Ling and P. J. H. Jones of the School of Dietetics and Human Nutrition, McGill University in Canada. (See the 1995 review of dietary phytosterols in *Life Sciences,* vol. 57, pp. 195–206.)

Among the possible additional benefits of products containing plant sterol extracts are the following:

- Phytosterols may help *decrease the risk for colon cancer* in both animals and humans. Ling and Jones report that dietary cholesterol has been implicated as a factor in colon cancer, especially through the work of strong bile acids in the intestinal tract (p. 203). To the extent that plant sterols can bind these bile acids, the risk of colon cancer may decrease.

● Plant sterols (sitosterols) may help the body *fight inflammation, hostile bacteria, and fungal conditions,* according to animal experiments cited by Ling and Jones.

● One type of sitosterol has been shown in animal experiments to fight heart disease through a mechanism other than lowering cholesterol. Specifically, *beta-sitosterol* has the power to *inhibit aggregation of blood platelets* and thus prevent the buildup of plaque and the clotting that may be key factors in cardiovascular disease.

● Another sitosterol chemical compound has demonstrated an *anti-ulcerative activity* when used in animals suffering from gastric ulcers.

Of course, more scientific research must be done in these areas to see whether the findings about animals will also apply to human populations. But up to this point, the research has been quite encouraging.

Question: Will it hurt me to have an occasional high-fat meal?

Answer: Just one high-fat meal can create real cardiovascular trouble.

Scientists from the University of Maryland School of Medicine actually found that a single high-fat meal will briefly reduce *endothelial function* of the blood vessels for up to four hours in healthy people with normal cholesterol levels. This term refers to the vessels' ability to expand and contract properly—and their tendency to become constricted and promote blockages to blood flow. (See *JAMA*, Nov. 26, 1997, pp. 1682–86.)

The participants, both men and women aged 24 to 54, ate one of three types of breakfasts:

1. a high-fat meal (900 calories, with 50 grams of fat—in other words, about half of the calories consumed were fat calories);

2. a low-fat meal (900 calories with zero fat); and

3. a high-fat meal—immediately before which they took two oral supplements: vitamin C (1 gram) and vitamin E (800 IU).

After these meals, the researchers checked the functioning of the brachial artery in the arm, at a point just above the elbow. They determined that there were no significant changes in artery function after the low-fat meal or the high-fat meal with vitamins.

But the investigators discovered a significant deterioration in the vessel's dilation function after the high-fat meal. In other words, there was more of a tendency for the artery to remain constricted—that is, not to dilate or expand.

The researchers speculated that the "hardening" of the vessel after the fatty breakfast probably resulted from the accumulation of lipoproteins rich in triglycerides. At the same time, they noted that taking vitamins C and E just before the meal could prevent any reduction in blood flow or blockage—perhaps through the protection of the blood lipids from oxidation by free radicals.

The first lesson I draw from this study is obvious: *Stay away from high-fat meals!*

The second, though not as self-evident, may be just as important: If you eat an occasional high-fat meal, *take large quantities of vitamins C and E* on a regular basis, but particularly before the meal.

Question: Is there any such thing as a "functional food drink" that will affect my cholesterol?

Answer: Yes. Drinks that may help your cholesterol include green tea and alcohol, consumed in moderate amounts. On the other hand, unfiltered coffee may hurt.

Green tea can lower "bad" LDL cholesterol and prevent it from turning into plaque deposits in vessels through oxidation, according to a review in *Bottom Line Health* (June 1998, p. 1). Total cholesterol levels averaged nine points lower in men who drank five cups of green tea than in those who didn't drink the beverage, according to one study.

Moderate alcohol consumption can decrease the risk of heart attack, according to a report in *The New England Journal of Medicine* (vol. 329, Dec. 16, 1993, pp. 1829–34).

Researchers from Harvard Medical School found that drinking one to three drinks of an alcoholic beverage can raise the levels of two subfractions of "good" HDL cholesterol, which is associated with lower cardiovascular risk. Specifically, the maximum effect on the HDL occurs with daily servings of one or two 12-ounce bottles of beer, or one or two 3.5-to-4-ounce glasses of wine, or one or two ordinary-size mixed drinks.

Many experts have cautioned, however, that other health problems increase significantly among those who regularly consume alcohol at these levels. Also, as I've warned in other contexts, to avoid raising the risk of hypertension (high blood pressure), breast cancer, and other diseases, it's wise for men to consume fewer than ten drinks per week, and women fewer than six drinks per week.

Unfiltered coffee can raise your cholesterol levels— though instant coffee and filtered coffee seem to have no negative effect. One 1997 Dutch study reported that unfiltered drinks such as espresso, French press, and Turkish coffee can raise "bad" LDL by an average of 5 percent. In this investigation, the participants drank five or more cups of unfiltered coffee per day. (See *New York Times,* June 13, 1997, p. A13.)

Question: How can stress affect my cholesterol?

Answer: It's long been known that stressful situations, including academic or occupational tests and high-pressure jobs, can result in an imbalance in cholesterol levels. But stress management can overcome many of these effects of stress, according to a report in the *Archives of Internal Medicine* (Oct. 27, 1997, pp. 2213–23).

In this study, investigators from the Duke University Medical Center found that cardiac patients who underwent stress management enjoyed a significantly lower risk of heart problems than did a control group or an exercise group. The stress-reduction group also had a slight but significant increase in their "good" HDL cholesterol and a decrease in their levels of triglycerides.

Question: I have a lot of trouble remembering to take my cholesterol medication. Sometimes I'll miss days at a time, especially when I forget to pick up my prescription. What kind of an effect is my forgetfulness having on my cholesterol?

Answer: You could be raising your risk for cardiovascular disease significantly—but unfortunately, you have a lot of company.

Only a quarter of patients with coronary artery disease are taking a cholesterol-lowering medication. This means that three-fourths of those in danger of a heart attack—and most heart attacks result from cholesterol-blocked coronary arteries—are not on the medications they need just to keep them alive!

There is more.

A 1998 study from Harvard, published in the *Journal of the American Medical Association,* revealed that patients who receive cholesterol drug prescriptions are likely not to have those prescriptions filled a significant part of the time. Specifically, the researchers determined that on average, for more than one-third of a year during which they were evaluated, the patients failed to fill their prescriptions. Even worse, after five years, about half of the surviving patients in the United States had stopped using the cholesterol-lowering drugs completely.

The main problem here is that there's a direct correlation between taking your pills and reducing your risk of cardiovascular disease. Many experts agree that being persistent in using prescribed cholesterol-controlling drugs will result in an estimated 39 percent reduction in cholesterol levels. But poor compliance will mean a decrease of only 11 percent. (See *JAMA,* May 13, 1998, p. 1461.)

Another research finding—which has a direct relationship to the functional foods we've been discussing in this book—is that only about half of all patients who should be on diet or drug therapy are receiving either of those treatments. This means people who should know better are unnecessarily putting themselves at a high risk for clogging of the arteries and a heart attack.

Why are so many patients failing to take advantage of these life-saving medications?

For one thing, research has confirmed that far too few doctors who should be prescribing cholesterol-lowering medications to patients who need them are actually doing so. In many cases, they just fail to recognize that a person with a stubborn cholesterol reading in the mid-200s may need a drug to bring his or her risk down to normal.

But the patients are also at fault. The investigators in the 1998 *JAMA* study noted that noncompliance may have occurred because some patients were dissatisfied with the drug they had been prescribed, perhaps due to unpleasant side effects or other problems.

For example, patients taking the statins, which have relatively few side effects, were more likely to stay with their regimen than were patients on bile acid sequestrants, which may produce more gastrointestinal difficulties.

Another quite obvious cause for noncompliance was simply that a significant proportion of those who received a doctor's prescription didn't have enough money to buy the prescribed medications. The researchers reported that poorer patients were only 58 percent as likely to continue with their drug therapy as those with higher incomes.

Finally, patients who had multiple cardiovascular risk factors—such as high blood pressure or diabetes in addition to elevated cholesterol—were more likely to take the drugs. Perhaps the reason was that they were motivated to stick with the medications because of exceptionally strong fears or concerns about their overall health.

What can you do if compliance with a prescription drug program is your stumbling block?

First, I'd suggest that you begin following a functional food strategy immediately if you haven't done so already. You may discover that you can lower your cholesterol enough this way to reduce your drugs significantly or eliminate them altogether.

Second, you might want to consult with your doctor about the possibility of switching to another drug.

Question: Can you summarize the main risk factors for cardiovascular disease—other than high or unbalanced cholesterol?

Answer: Here they are in a quick checklist:

- **High blood pressure.** To be in the healthiest range—and the lowest risk category for heart disease—most people should have a systolic (upper) reading of 130 or below, and a diastolic (lower) reading reading of 83 or below.

- **Personal history of heart attack or bypass or other cardiovascular surgery.** If you've suffered from heart or vessel disease once, you're much more likely to have the problem again.

- **Family history of heart attack.** You're more likely to have heart trouble if either or both of your parents suffered from a heart attack before age 60 and especially before age 50.

- **Smoking.** If you smoked on a daily or regular basis within the past year, your cardiovascular risk went up significantly.

- **Stress.** If you experience moderate to intense anxiety and stress in your daily life, your risk for heart attack or other cardiovascular disease increases considerably.

- **Diabetes or high blood glucose levels.** Remember that the desired glucose range on a standard blood test is 80 to 120 mg/dl.

- **Your age.** If you're under 30, your age places you in a low-risk category. Every decade you grow older, your risk of cardiovascular disease increases progressively. It begins to level off after you pass your sixties.

- **Percent of body fat.** The low-risk body-fat range for men is 19 percent of total body weight or lower, and for women is 22 percent or lower.

Question: I have close-to-normal cholesterol and no other significant cardiovascular risk factors. Is there any point in my taking functional foods to lower my blood lipids still further?

Answer: The dramatic recent advances in cholesterol and blood-lipid research have caused scientists and practicing physicians alike to consider whether to extend treatments to people who were once considered normal or healthy.

Their reasoning sometimes goes like this: If there is even a slight chance that a person may suffer or die from cardiovascular disease, why not do what you can to eliminate all risk?

One of the most important recent studies that has confirmed the benefits of treating healthy people with slightly above average cholesterol levels focused on one of the statin drugs produced by Merck & Company, lovastatin (Mevacor). The study, conducted by John R. Downs, M.D., and colleagues, Wilford Hall Medical Center, Lackland Air Force Base, San Antonio (AFCAPS/TexCAPS), was published in 1998 in *JAMA*.

The investigation involved more than 6,600 middle-aged and elderly men and women with average cholesterol levels, who were divided into a drug-using group and a placebo group. After taking the pills for five years, those with the lovastatin had 37 percent fewer heart attacks and other signs of cardiovascular disease than did the participants on the dummy pill. (See *New York Times,* May 27, 1998, p. 1.)

The participants had no history or diagnosis of heart disease, and their average total cholesterol was 221, a figure that put them in the fifty-first percentile for all Americans. Also, their "bad" LDL cholesterol level before the treatments began was 150 mg/dl—a measurement that placed them only 10 points above the average for American adults. On the other hand, their "good" HDL cholesterol levels were rather low at the start: 36 for the men and 40 for the women.

At the end of the study, the group that took the lovastatin experienced a 25 percent, 35-point drop in their "bad" LDL cholesterol and a 6 percent rise in their "good" HDL cholesterol.

To sum up these results, it seems that apparently healthy people with average or slightly elevated levels of total cholesterol—but relatively low levels of "good" HDL cholesterol—can benefit from going on drug therapy. On the other hand, this kind of prevention can be expensive. An editorial in the same issue of *JAMA* pointed out that the annual cost of drugs for the lovastatin group ranged from $1,075 to $1,766.

Is the price worth the prevention?

I would never put a price tag on saving a person's health or life—and your physician, looking at your entire cardiovascular risk profile, may decide that you are candidate for treatment. But I would strongly recommend that before turning to drugs, patients with slightly high total or LDL cholesterol, or a low level of "good" HDL cholesterol (with an out-of-balance cholesterol ratio), should first try the nondrug route.

An illustration of this approach involved 50-year-old Ron, who had nearly normal cholesterol readings but still felt there was room for improvement.

At the start, his total cholesterol was 192, or well within the "acceptable" risk range. Also, Ron's "bad" LDL was an acceptable 127. But his "good" HDL was 42, and that gave him a ratio of 4.57. Both of these latter readings placed him in "borderline" risk categories.

Ron tried a plant stanol margarine for eight weeks and found that his total cholesterol dropped to 180, and his LDL went down to 114. His HDL stayed the same at 42—with the result that he ended up with a ratio of 4.28, which was at the edge of the "acceptable" risk category.

Was it worth it for Ron to try to fine-tune his lipids with functional foods, given his relatively low risk before he began the study?

I'm sympathetic to his approach because research increasingly suggests that the total cholesterol "healthy" ceiling of 200 should actually be lower for most people—below 180 if possible. With no danger of side effects from the functional foods, it would seem that a person in Ron's position would have everything to gain and nothing to lose by trying them.

Question: Will lowering my cholesterol really prolong my life?

Answer: As early as 1990, representatives of the American Heart Association and the National Heart, Lung and Blood Institute responded with a strong yes.

They put it this way in the official AHA journal *Circulation* (vol. 81, no. 5, May 1990, pp. 1721–33): "Evidence from epidemiologic studies strongly suggests that low serum (blood) cholesterol levels are accompanied by prolongation of life."

These experts noted that "reduction in total mortality . . . was reported in three recent clinical studies"—the

Coronary Drug Project, the Oslo Study Diet and Antismoking Trial, and the Stockholm Ischemic Heart Disease Study.

In addition, they wanted to go on record with answers to these two related questions: "Is high serum cholesterol a risk factor for coronary heart disease?" and "Will lowering serum cholesterol help prevent coronary heart disease?"

They responded unequivocally: "Strong scientific data provide positive answers to both of these questions."

Finally, in emphasizing the benefits of lowering cholesterol, they went beyond the question of mortality. They noted that critics who had doubted the importance of reducing elevated cholesterol had been so preoccupied with death that they had overlooked the impact on the quality of life:

> *"Approximately 5 million Americans are living and suffering from CHD [coronary heart disease]. By decreasing this number, the quality of life for millions of Americans can be improved, regardless of whether they live longer. Thus, an important goal of a cholesterol reduction program should be to prevent CHD and, by doing so, improve the quality of life."*

These conclusions represent relatively early statements by the world's best medical minds on the importance of lowering even slightly elevated cholesterol. Since that time, our knowledge has increased dramatically, as landmark research reports have confirmed again and again that high or unbalanced cholesterol is a killer.

I won't repeat other studies I've cited throughout these pages, including a flood of research demonstrating that life can be prolonged and health improved by lowering cholesterol with the new statin drugs.

Nor will I go into detail again about the studies showing the benefits of lifestyle changes, such as low-fat diets and regular exercise.

I merely cite the above conclusion to make it absolutely clear how the leading experts on cholesterol feel—and have felt for nearly a decade—about the importance of lowering or balancing your cholesterol.

So if anyone tries to tell you that "there's a lot of confusion on this subject" or "research is inconclusive," just refer them to the succinct but powerful statements in the above report. And use these official conclusions and recommendations to motivate yourself to make better use of lifestyle adjustments and functional foods to improve your own blood-lipid profile.

13

Our Nutriceutical Future

We live in highly exciting times, as the fields of medicine and nutrition converge before our very eyes—and present us with far greater potential to exercise control not only over our cholesterol but over our health as a whole.

Yet as we move further into the functional food era, we must be prepared for surprises along the way. I encounter them practically every day, as I counsel patients who use not only the traditional medicine we offer at the Cooper Clinic but also less conventional approaches to prevention and treatment.

One of those surprises involved Rob, an entrepreneur in his mid-fifties who had been my patient for nearly twenty years. By most standards, Rob seemed to be doing everything right as far as his health was concerned, and up to this point, he had shown no signs or symptoms of heart disease.

Several exercise stress tests he had taken, including one within the previous year, had resulted in completely normal electrocardiograms and an excellent aerobic fitness rating. Also, he had normal blood pressure and was in a low range for his age for most other cardiovascular risk factors.

But Rob's cholesterol measurements were an exception—which he had been unable to overcome completely with his diet and exercise.

A recent blood test showed that his total cholesterol was 201 and his HDL was 39—results that gave him a ratio of 5.2. His "bad" LDL was 143. These cholesterol readings were all "borderline" according to chart 1 on page 30—a result that we both knew he should try to improve if he could.

Because it was inappropriate to consider prescription medications at this stage with Rob, we agreed that it wouldn't hurt to give functional foods a try. So he got three bottles of the Benecol salad dressing, including the ranch and thousand island preparations.

One thing Rob particularly liked about the functional food was that he could fit it into his daily meal plan easily, without having to upset his carefully structured diet. All that was required was for him to substitute the Benecol salad dressing for other low-fat and no-fat brands he was using.

Because Rob had stocked up with limited amounts of the dressing as a kind of "trial run," he decided to take only two-thirds of the recommended amount per day. This meant that he would take in less than 2 grams per day of the plant stanol, even though the usual dose is 3 to 4.5 grams. (If he had consulted me about this decision, I would have advised him to take the full "dose" because that's the only way you can get the full benefit—but he didn't.)

At the end of a 16-day period, Rob ran out of the salad dressing and immediately scheduled a blood test. The results were not at all what either of us had expected.

First of all, Rob's total cholesterol actually went up slightly, to 205, but his "bad" LDL cholesterol went down to 135—a 6 percent drop.

The most startling result, however, was that his "good"

HDL cholesterol actually went up to 51—an incredible 31 percent increase that gave him the highest reading he had reached in nearly 20 years of testing! As a result, Rob achieved the best ratio of his entire life—a 4.0, which placed him for the first time in his life in the "acceptable" risk category. A second set of blood tests confirmed the dramatic improvement.

What had happened here?

The reduction in "bad" LDL cholesterol was fairly predictable. The decrease was lower than the average in most research studies, but Rob had taken a lower dose that what was recommended.

The surprising rise in the "good" HDL cholesterol, which did wonders for Rob's ratio, seems to have involved a special individual biological reaction that the nutriceutical produced in his body. Some people who take Benecol do see their HDL levels go up, though not enough experience this benefit to make it statistically significant. Rob apparently happened to be one of the lucky ones.

Rob's experience remains particularly important to me because it highlights the fact that we must be prepared for many unexpected twists and turns as we enjoy these fast-moving adventures in health that lie just ahead of us.

It's easy for a traditional practicing physician like me to become a little disconcerted when I see a stubborn problem like Rob's ratio resolved in record time through something as simple and ordinary as a salad dressing. But I'm learning, as are many of my colleagues, that the best medical practice in these unusual times demands that we expect the unexpected and accept surprise as the rule, not the exception.

The most effective healers of every era have tested new ground, searched new horizons, and released their full reservoirs of creativity. Today the challenge is nutriceuticals. But I'm already looking forward to what tomorrow will bring.

Glossary

Anticholesterol. A term sometimes used to refer to those chemically produced plant stanol and plant sterol extracts that are able to lower total and "bad" LDL cholesterol levels.

Antioxidants. Chemical agents, including certain vitamins (such as E and C) and minerals (like selenium), that are able to combat or neutralize *free radicals,* or unstable oxygen molecules in the body. Sometimes called *free radical scavengers,* these antioxidants help prevent the oxidation of "bad" LDL cholesterol in the blood and the subsequent development of atherosclerosis.

ApoB. A short term for Apolipoprotein B.

Apolipoprotein B. The protein component of the LDL molecule, which many experts feel provides the best indication of the amount of "bad" LDL cholesterol circulating in the bloodstream. Also, a high amount of ApoB in the blood may signal a high risk for development of atherosclerosis, or vessel disease.

Arteriosclerosis. A word often used interchangeably with *atherosclerosis* to mean hardening of the arteries, or clogging of the vessels. (*Arteriosclerosis* comes from a Greek word meaning "hardness.") Technically, atherosclerosis—which is the more precise medical term for the buildup of plaque in blood vessels—is a type of arteriosclerosis.

Atherosclerosis. Often used synonymously with *arte-*

riosclerosis to mean the vessel disease that involves hardening of the inner lining of the arteries through the buildup of plaque. Plaque occurs as oxidized LDL cholesterol sticks to the vessel walls and builds up gradually to close the opening (lumen) through which blood flows. Atherosclerosis is the main cause of cardiovascular disease, heart attacks, and strokes.

"Bad" cholesterol. A popular term for low-density lipoprotein or LDL cholesterol. Research has linked this subcomponent of cholesterol to the oxidation process that leads to the buildup of plaque and the blockage (occlusion) of the arteries.

Bile acid. An emulsifier—or agent controlling the suspension of one liquid in another—which assists with fat and cholesterol absorption. Bile acids are important in the production of micelles, the "vehicles" in the intestine that enable cholesterol to be absorbed into the bloodstream through the intestinal wall.

The bile contains most of the body's cholesterol that eventually enters the bloodstream through the intestinal wall. Certain functional foods and drugs that interfere with bile acid synthesis can prevent cholesterol from reentering the bloodstream.

Bile acid sequestrant drugs. A class of cholesterol-lowering prescription medications that operate by "binding" or turning into waste bile acids that contain cholesterol as they return from the liver to the intestinal tract. Common drugs in this class include cholestyramine (Questran and Questran Light) and colestipol (Colestid).

Canola oil. A type of rapeseed oil that is low in saturated fats and high in monounsaturated fats. (Common in Europe, the rape plant is an herb from the mustard family.)

Cardiovascular disease. Disease of the heart and blood vessels, especially atherosclerosis. Also called CVD.

Cholesterol. A blood fat or lipid that circulates in the blood and consists of many different subcomponents—such as low-density lipoprotein (LDL) and high-density lipoprotein (HDL). Cholesterol is now regarded as a main factor in the development of atherosclerosis and coronary heart disease.

Cholesterol risk. The degree to which out-of-control cholesterol affects overall cardiovascular risk—or risk of heart and vessel disease. Cardiovascular risk goes up with high total cholesterol, high LDL cholesterol, low HDL cholesterol, or a high ratio of total to HDL cholesterol.

Cholestin. A Chinese red yeast rice—also known as hongqu, hong qu, or hung-chu—that has shown the ability to lower cholesterol. It is similar to the drug lovastatin (marketed under the brand name Mevacor).

Coronary artery disease. Atherosclerosis or clogging of the coronary arteries that supply blood to the heart muscle. Also referred to as CAD.

Coronary heart disease. Also called *ischemic heart disease,* this condition involves the inadequate supply of blood and oxygen to the heart because of blockage of a coronary artery. Heart tissue dies when the blood supply is shut off. Also referred to as CHD.

Esterification. A chemical process that combines fatty acids with plant sterols or stanols to increase solubility and make it possible to include the plant extracts in ordinary foods.

Estrogen. The female hormone that has a protective effect before menopause in keeping total cholesterol and LDL cholesterol low, and HDL cholesterol high.

Fibrates, Fibric acid derivatives. A class of cholesterol-controlling medications that lower triglycerides, raise "good" HDL cholesterol, lower total cholesterol, and sometimes reduce "bad" LDL. An example is gemfibrozil (Lopid).

Folic acid. A member of the B-vitamin complex family. Lowers blood levels of homocysteine, an amino acid product that has been linked to vessel disease.

Free radical. Unstable oxygen molecules that cause oxidation of "bad" LDL cholesterol in the blood—a process that is central to the development of blockages in the vessels.

Functional food. A popular term referring to foods that have the power to improve or prevent health conditions and diseases. They may be *designed* (foods containing additives produced through a chemical process) or *traditional* (foods without such additives). Also called *nutriceuticals* or *nutraceuticals.*

"Good" cholesterol. A popular term for high-density lipoprotein (HDL), which has been linked to protection from atherosclerosis.

Hardening of the arteries. A popular term for atherosclerosis and arteriosclerosis. The process of atherosclerosis is associated with plaque that hardens the *intima,* or inner lining of the arteries.

HDL cholesterol. High-density lipoprotein, a subcomponent of total cholesterol. High levels have been associated with greater protection from cardiovascular disease. A key part of the ratio of total cholesterol to HDL cholesterol.

Homocysteine. A product of the breakdown of the amino acid methionine in the body. High levels in the blood are associated with a higher risk of cardiovascular disease.

Hormone replacement therapy. A treatment for postmenopausal women that involves a combination of estrogen and progestin. Among other things, this therapy is used to bring cholesterol into balance. Also known as HRT. Also sometimes referred to as *estrogen replacement therapy* (ERT).

HRT. (*See* **Hormone replacement therapy.**)

Hypercholesterolemia. A condition characterized by an abnormally large amount of cholesterol in the blood. Also called *hypercholesteremia.*

Hyperlipidemia. A condition involving an excess level of fats or lipids in the blood, including cholesterol, triglycerides, and various lipoproteins.

Hypertriglyceridemia. High blood levels of the lipid triglycerides.

Insoluble fiber. A stringy plant component, found in such foods as wheat bran, that won't dissolve in water.

Ischemia. An inability to get enough blood and oxygen to a tissue, such as the heart. Eventually, ischemia can produce death.

LDL cholesterol. Low-density lipoprotein. A subcomponent of cholesterol, often referred to as "bad" cholesterol.

Lipids. Fat or fatlike particles in the body and blood.

Lipoprotein(a), Lp(a). A subfraction of cholesterol. It is sometimes known as "ugly cholesterol" because of reports linking it to a very high risk of heart and vessel disease.

mg/dl. Milligrams per deciliter—the common unit of measurement, in the United States, for blood lipids such as cholesterol and triglycerides.

mmol/dl. Millimoles per deciliter—the common unit of measurement, in Europe, for blood lipids. To translate *mmol/dl* into *mg/dl,* multiply the *mmol/dl* figure by 38.7.

Micelle. A tiny, fatty droplet formed from the bile in the small intestine. Micelles serve as the "carts" that convey cholesterol through the intestinal wall into the bloodstream.

Monounsaturated fats. A "healthy" fat characterized

chemically by one unsaturated link or double bond in the carbon chain. Foods that have high amounts of this fat include olive oil and canola oil. Also referred to as a MUFA.

Myocardial infarction (MI). Heart attack.

Niacin. An over-the-counter vitamin B_3 product, which can be a powerful treatment to lower total and "bad" LDL cholesterol without lowering "good" HDL cholesterol. But this drug should be taken only under the supervision of a physician because of the possibility of liver damage, especially with high doses. Time-release capsules aren't recommended. Also called *nicotinic acid.*

Nicotinic acid. *See* **Niacin.**

Nutriceutical (nutraceutical). Another name for functional food. For a discussion of spelling variations, see the author's note.

Occlusion. A blockage or shutting off, as with a narrowed artery or artery blocked by a blood clot.

Oxidation. Combining of oxygen with other molecules or elements. Rust is a form of oxidation, as is the spoiling of food through rancidity. LDL cholesterol is sometimes said to "rust" or "go rancid" when free radicals cause oxidation of LDL in the blood vessels.

Oxidative stress. The process of deterioration that occurs through oxidation.

Phytostanol. Plant stanol, which is the fully saturated form of phytosterols (a component of vegetable fats and oils).

Phytosterol. Plant sterol, which is a natural component of vegetable fats and oils. It closely resembles cholesterol in molecular structure.

Phytosterolemia. An extremely rare condition where the

body actually absorbs plant sterols rather than rejecting them. This disease can result in premature atherosclerosis if too many phytosterols get through the intestinal wall and into the bloodstream.

Plant stanol. *See* **Phytostanol.**

Plant stanol ester. A chemically prepared plant stanol that is soluble in fat and can be combined with many different types of foods. A stanol is a fully saturated form of a sterol.

Plant sterol. *See* **Phytosterol**.

Plaque. A yellow, swollen area on the inner wall of an artery, caused by the buildup of fatty deposits—primarily oxidized LDL cholesterol.

Plasma. Fluid part of blood, without red and white blood cells.

Polyunsaturated fats. A fatty acid found in many foods that has more than one unsaturated link in the carbon chain. Foods with high amounts of this fat include corn, soybeans, and safflower. Also referred to as PUFA.

Psyllium. A soluble-fiber grain that has been shown to lower cholesterol. For the grain's operation as a functional food, the psyllium-husk seeds are the operable part. It is found in some popular cereals.

Rapeseed oil. A vegetable oil with high concentrations of the monounsaturated fatty acid oleic acid. Also known as *canola oil.*

Ratio. With cholesterol, refers to the ratio of total cholesterol to good cholesterol. A high ratio indicates high risk, and a low ratio, low risk.

Saturated fats. Fats most often associated with a higher risk of high cholesterol and cardiovascular disease. They are characterized chemically by single bonds in an organic molecule. Saturated fats tend to stay hard at room temperature, while unsaturated fats are more liquid.

Serum. The yellowish part of whole blood remaining after blood has clotted.

Sitostanol. A type of plant stanol, which is a saturated form of a sterol.

Sitosterol. A type of plant sterol, which is a natural component of vegetable fats and oils.

Soluble fiber. Plant fibers, found in foods like oats, psyllium, and apples, that dissolve in water or in the body's environment. These fibers have been associated with lowering cholesterol.

Statin drugs. These HMG-CoA reductase inhibitors lower cholesterol by preventing synthesis of "bad" LDL cholesterol in the liver. They also help the body remove LDL from the blood by stimulating LDL "receptors," which "hook" LDL in the blood and neutralize it. Statins are more effective than most other types of cholesterol-lowering drugs currently on the market, and they have relatively few side effects. But they have been associated with some liver problems, so liver function must be monitored regularly.

Stress test. A fitness and heart-function test that requires the patient to exercise to maximum capacity on a stationary bicycle or treadmill, while being monitored with an electrocardiogram.

Trans fats. Trans fats, often listed as *hydrogenated* or *partially hydrogenated* on food labels, are formed by a chemical process that hardens vegetable oils to prevent them from spoiling.

These fats—which make up about 3 percent of fats in the average diet—are also often called *hidden fats*. The reason is that they lurk unheralded in a wide variety of products, including stick margarine, cookies, crackers, and other commercially baked goods. Yet trans fats may be the most dangerous fats of all in fostering the buildup of plaque in the arteries. (See *New England Journal of Medicine,* Nov. 20, 1997.)

Triglycerides. The main fat in foods, and a common lipid in the bloodstream. Associated recently with a significantly increased risk of heart disease.

Ultrafast CT scan. A computer-imaging device, produced by the Imatron company, that can detect calcification of arteries as well as other internal problems.

Vitamin C. An antioxidant that has been linked to lower cholesterol.

Vitamin E (natural). A powerful antioxidant that is associated with lower oxidation of LDL cholesterol and other cardiovascular benefits. The natural version is often listed on labels as *d-alpha tocopherol.*

VLDL cholesterol. Very low-density lipoprotein, a subcomponent of total cholesterol that is linked to the transport of triglycerides and other lipids in the bloodstream.

About the Author

Kenneth H. Cooper, M.D., M.P.H., is recognized internationally as the "father of aerobics" and the leading spokesman for the preventive medicine movement.

A graduate of the University of Oklahoma School of Medicine and the Harvard University School of Public Health, he introduced the term *aerobics* to the world with his bestseller *Aerobics.* Soon after publication of this major work, he founded the Cooper Clinic, the Cooper Aerobics Center, and the Cooper Institute for Aerobics Research in Dallas. Landmark scientific studies have regularly emerged from the huge database and research facilities at the institute in Dallas.

During his career, Dr. Cooper has authored sixteen books, which have sold more than 30 million copies in over forty languages. These include *The Aerobics Program for Total Well-Being, Aerobics for Women* (with Mildred Cooper), *The Antioxidant Revolution, Preventing Osteoporosis, Overcoming Hypertension, Kid Fitness,* and the bestseller *Controlling Cholesterol.*

Index